CBS Confident Pharmacy Series

Pharmaceutics I

Third Edition

for First Year Diploma in Pharmacy

(0805) Strictly Based on Syllabus as per ER1991

Question–Answer Type Notes and Board Question Papers (1995 to 2017)

Salient Features

❏ Total Confidence and 100 percent Success in Every Examination.

❏ Repeatedly Asked Board Questions Indicated in Brackets.

❏ Chapterwise Collection of Very Important Questions.

❏ Written in Very Simple and Lucid Language.

❏ Board Question Papers 2015–2017 given at the End of Text.

CBS Confident Pharmacy Series

Pharmaceutics I

Third Edition

for First Year Diploma in Pharmacy

(**0805**) Strictly Based on Syllabus as per ER1991

V.N. Raje M Pharm

Principal
Gourishankar Education Society's
GES College of Pharmacy (D Pharm)
Limb, Satara, Maharashtra

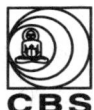

CBS

CBS Publishers & Distributors Pvt Ltd

New Delhi • Bengaluru • Chennai • Kochi • Kolkata • Mumbai
Bhopal • Bhubaneswar • Hyderabad • Jharkhand • Nagpur • Patna • Pune
• Uttarakhand • Dhaka (Bangladesh) • Kathmandu (Nepal)

Pharmaceutics I
Third Edition

ISBN: 978-93-86478-48-1

Third Edition: 2018
   Reprint: 2018, 2019, 2020, 2021
First Edition: 2010
   Reprint: 2011
Second Edition: 2015
   Reprint: 2016

Published by Satish Kumar Jain and produced by Varun Jain for

CBS Publishers & Distributors Pvt Ltd
4819/XI Prahlad Street, 24 Ansari Road, Daryaganj, New Delhi 110 002, India
Ph: 011-23289259, 23266861, 23266867   Website: www.cbspd.com
Fax: 011-23243014   e-mail: delhi@cbspd.com; cbspubs@airtelmail.in
Corporate Office: 204 FIE, Industrial Area, Patparganj, Delhi 110 092
Ph: 011-49344934   e-mail: publishing@cbspd.com; publicity@cbspd.com
Fax: 011-49344935

Branches

- **Bengaluru:** Seema House, 2975, 17th Cross, K.R. Road,
  Banasankari 2nd Stage, Bengaluru 560 070, Karnataka
  Ph: +91-80-26771678/79   Fax: +91-80-26771680   e-mail: bangalore@cbspd.com
- **Chennai:** 7, Subbaraya Street, Shenoy Nagar, Chennai 600 030, Tamil Nadu
  Ph: +91-44-26680620, 26681266   Fax: +91-44-42032115   e-mail: chennai@cbspd.com
- **Kochi:** 68/1534, 35, 36, Power House Road, Opp. KSEB, Kochi 682018, Kerala
  Ph: +91-484-4059061-65   Fax: +91-484-4059065   e-mail: kochi@cbspd.com
- **Kolkata:** 6/B, Ground Floor, Rameswar Shaw Road, Kolkata-700 014, West Bengal
  Ph: +91-33-22891126, 22891127, 22891128   e-mail: kolkata@cbspd.com
- **Mumbai:** 83-C, Dr E Moses Road, Worli, Mumbai-400018, Maharashtra
  Ph: +91-22-24902340/41   Fax: +91-22-24902342   e-mail: mumbai@cbspd.com

Representatives

Bhopal	0-8319310552	Bhubaneswar	0-9911037372	Hyderabad	0-9885175004
Jharkhand	0-9811541605	Nagpur	0-9421945513	Patna	0-9334159340
Pune	0-9623451994	Uttarakhand	0-9716462459	Dhaka (Bangladesh)	01912-003485
Kathmandu (Nepal)	977-9818742655				

Printed at Mudrak, Noida, UP, India

to

my beloved family

Preface to the Third Edition

The third edition of the now popular and successful book includes Board Question Papers 1995 to 2017. The book has been written to meet the requirements of students of Diploma in Pharmacy (D Pharm) in accordance with the new revised syllabus ER1991 prescribed by Pharmacy Council of India.

This book is small and humble effort has been put in for compiling necessary information on the subject. An attempt has been made to demystify and simplify the basic concepts for the students of pharmacy and to enable them get an evergreen success in MSBTE examinations.

The salient features of the present book are:

- Lucid and easy language,
- To the point answers,
- Remembering facts in the simplest way, and
- Infusing confidence in the reader to appear in the Board Examinations.

Hence the series is named

CBS Confident Pharmacy Series

I am confident that this book will be useful to both the students and the teachers of Diploma in Pharmacy as well as the candidates desiring to succeed in competitive examinations for better job opportunities in pharmacy profession such as hospital pharmacists in PHCs, civil hospitals, etc.

Raje Vijay N

Acknowledgements

I express my heartfelt thanks to Prof Madan Jagtap, Chairman, Gourishankar Education Society, Satara Maharashtra, for consistent encouragement and inspiration for writing this book.

I wish to acknowledge the prompt and efficient help given by Prof Milind Jagtap, Mr Jaywant Salunkhe, Mr Appa Rajage, Mr Nitin Mudalgikar, and Mr Shrirang Katekar of Gourishankar Education Society, Satara.

I am also thankful to Shri Satish Kumar Jain, Chairman and Managing Director, and Shri RN Mandal, General Manager, Pune Branch, CBS Publishers & Distributors Pvt Ltd, for their sustained efforts and keen interest in the publication of this book.

I wish all my beloved students to have a great success in the Board Examinations.

Raje Vijay N

Syllabus

(As per ER 1991)

Pharmaceutics I

1. Introduction of different dosage forms. Their classification with examples—their relative applications. Familiarisation with new drug delivery systems.
2. Introduction to Pharmacopoeias with special reference to the Indian Pharmacopoeia.
3. Metrology-systems of weights and measures—Calculations including conversion from one to another system, percentage calculations and adjustment of products use of alligation method in calculations isotonic solutions.
4. Packaging of Pharmaceuticals—Desirable features of a container, types of containers. Study of glass and plastics as materials for containers and rubber as material for closures, their merits and demerits. Introduction to aerosol packaging.
5. Size reduction—Objectives, and factors affecting size reduction. Methods of size reduction-study of Hammer mill, Ball mill, Fluid energy mill and disintegrator.
6. Size separation—Size separation by sifting, official standards for powders. Sedimentation methods of size separation. Construction and working of Cyclone separator.
7. Mixing and Homogenisation—Liquid mixing and powder mixing, mixing of semisolids. Study of silverson mixer—Homogeniser; Planetary mixer; Agitated powder mixer; Triple roller mill; Propeller mixer, Colloid mill and Hand homogeniser. Double cone mixer.
8. Filtration and Clarification—Theory of filtration, filter media; Filter aids and selection of filters, Study of the following filtration equipment—Filter press, Sintered filters, Filter candles, Metafilter.
9. Extraction and Galenicals—(a) Study of percolation and meceration and their modification, continuous hot extracrion.

Applications in the preparation of tinctures and extracts. (b) Introduction to Ayurvedic dosage forms.

10. Heat processes, Evaporation—Definition, Factors affecting evaporation, Study of evaporating still and Evaporating pan.

11. Distillation—Simple distillation and Fractional distillation; Steam distillation and vacuum distillation. Study of vacuum still, preparation of purified water IP and water for Injection IP. Construction and working of the still used for the same.

12. Introduction to drying processes—Study of tray dryers; Fluidized bed dryer, Vacuum dryer and Freeze dryer.

13. Sterilization—Concept of sterilization and its differences from disinfection, Thermal resistance of micro-organisms. Detailed study of the following sterilization processes.
    (i) Sterilization with moist heat
    (ii) Dry heat sterilization
    (iii) Sterilization by radiation
    (iv) Sterilization filtration and
    (v) Gaseous sterilization.
    Aseptic techniques—Application of sterilization processes in hospitals particularly with reference to surgical dressings and intravenous fluids. Precautions for safe and effective handling of sterilization equipment.

14. Processing of Tablets—Definition; Different types of compressed tablets and their properties. Processes involved in the production of tablets; Tablets excipients; Defects in tablets; Evaluation of tablets; Physical standards including Disintegration and dissolution. Tablet coating, Sugar coating, Film coating, Enteric coating and microencapsulation (Tablet coating may be dealt in an elementary manner).

15. Processing of Capsules—Hard and soft gelatin capsules; different sizes of capsules; filling of capsules; handling and storage of capsules. Special applications of capsules.

16. Study of immunological products like sera, vaccines, toxoids and their preparations.

Contents

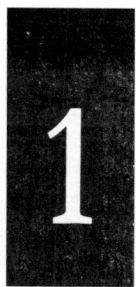

Introduction to Dosage Forms

1 Define the following:

☞ **1. Drug (W. 96, 98, 04, 07, 08)**

"Drug is a substance used for the diagnosis, treatment, mitigation or prevention of diseases in the human beings or animals and they may be used internally or externally."

2. Additives

"The nondrugs components which are mixed with drug to form a suitable dosage form is called additives or adjuvants or exipients."

3. Dose

"It is the quantity of drug required to produce the desired action."

4. Dosage Form (S. 06; W. 96, 98, 04, 07, 08)

"The drug is combined with nondrug component (additives) and the resulting form of drug is known as dosage form."

2 Give importance of dosage forms. Why are dosage forms required? (S. 09; W. 00)

☞ Dosage forms are required because:
- To protect the drug from oxidation, hydrolysis and reduction.
- To provide a safe and convenient delivery of accurate dosage.

1

- To mask the bitter, salty taste and odour of a drug.
- To provide optimum drug action through inhalation, e.g. aerosols.
- To provide maximum drug action.
- To provide sustained release action.
- To protect the drug from destructive effect of gastric juice.
- To provide the drugs within body tissues, e.g. injections.

3 Give two examples of the following additives (pharmaceutical aids). (S. 99; W. 96)

☞ 1. Diluents: Lactose, sucrose.
2. Binders: Acacia, gelatin.
3. Lubricants: Talc, magnesium stearate.
4. Disintegrants: Starch, cellulose.
5. Adsorbents: Bentonite, magnesium silicate.
6. Glidants: Talc, magnesium stearate.
7. Granulating agents: Water, alcohol.
8. Humectants: Glycerin, sorbitol.
9. Colouring agents: Amarnath, indigocarmine.
10. Flavouring agents: Lemon grass oil, menthal oil, peppermint oil.
11. Sweeteners: Saccharin, sucrose, dextrose.

4 Give classification of dosage forms. (S. 96, 01, 06; W. 03, 04, 06)

☞

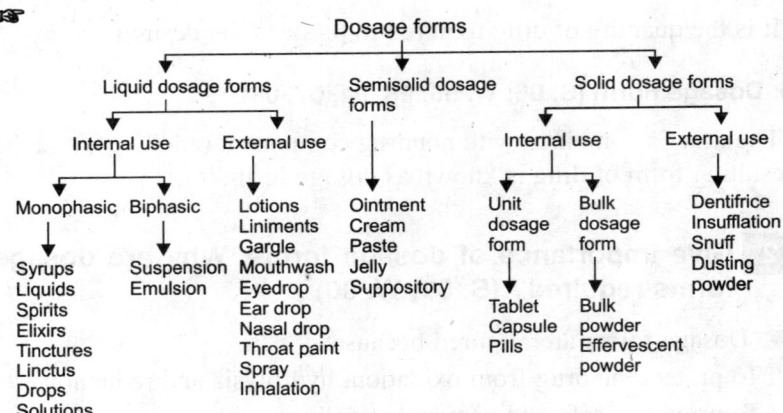

5 Define the terms.

☞ **1. Syrups:** Syrups are sweet, viscous concentrated aqueous solutions of sucrose or other sugars.

2. Elixirs: Elixirs are clear, pleasantly flavoured, sweetened hydroalcoholic liquid preparations for oral use.

3. Spirits (essences): Spirits are alcoholic or hydroalcoholic solutions of volatile substances.

4. Tinctures: Tinctures are alcoholic or hydroalcoholic solutions of vegetable drugs.

5. Linctus: Linctus are viscous, liquid preparations containing sucrose and medicinal agent and are used for the relief of cough.

6. Mixture: Mixture is the liquid medicine for internal use containing several doses in one bettle.

7. Draught: Draught is the liquid medicine for internal use containing single dose in one bottle.

8. Solutions: Solutions are liquid preparations containing one or more chemical substances dissolved in water.

9. Emulsion: Emulsion is a biphasic system containing two immiscible liquids, in which one liquid is distributed in other in the form of minute globules and the system is being stabilised by addition of third substance known as emulsifying agent.

10. Suspension: Suspension is a biphasic system in which solid substances are suspended in a liquid medium and the system is stabilised by addition of suspending agent.

11. Lotions: Lotions are fluid preparations which are applied to the skin without friction.

12. Liniments: Liniments are fluid preparations applied externally to the skin with friction.

13. Gargles: Gargles are aqueous solutions of drug used to treat, throat infections, usually supplied in concentrated form.

14. Mouthwashes: Mouthwashes are aqueous solutions of the drugs used to wash the mouth cavity and deodorise the mouth cavity.

15. Throat paint: These are viscous preparations applied to the mucous membrane of throat with the help of soft brush.

16. Eye lotions: These are aqueous solutions of drugs used to clean and wash the eyes.

17. **Ear drops:** These are solutions of drugs which are instilled into the ear cavity with the help of dropper.
18. **Nasal drops:** These are solutions of drugs which are instilled into the nasal cavity with the help of dropper.
19. **Inhalations:** Inhalations are solutions of volatile substances administered by the nasal route in the form of vapours.
20. **Lozenges:** Lozenges are solid preparations containing sugar and gums and are used to medicate the mouth and throat.
21. **Ointments:** Ointments are semisolid preparations intended for external application to the skin or mucous membrane.
22. **Creams:** Creams are viscous emulsions for external applications to the skin or mucous membrane.
23. **Paste:** Pastes are semisolid preparations for external application containing a large amount of finely powdered solids.
24. **Jellies:** Jellies are transparent or translucent semisolid preparations for external application.
25. **Suppositories:** These are solid bodies, suitably shaped for insertion into the rectum.
26. **Pessaries:** These are solid bodies, suitably shaped for insertion into the vaginal cavity.
27. **Tablets:** Tablets are solid, flat or biconvex disc-shaped, prepared by compressing a drug or mixture of drugs with or without diluents.
28. **Capsules:** It is a solid unit dosage form usually containing powdered drug enclosed within the water soluble gelatin shell.
29. **Pills:** These are small rounded solid dosage forms containing medicaments.
30. **Insufflations:** Insufflations are medicated dusting powders which are blown into the body cavities like nose, ear, throat with the help of an insufflator.
31. **Snuffs:** Snuffs are finely divided powdered dosage forms of medicament which are inhaled into nostrils for their decongestion action.
32. **Dentrifices:** These are the preparations in the form of toothpaste or tooth powder which are used for cleansing the teeth.
33. **Plasters:** Plasters are solid preparations of external applications which adhere to skin and keep a dressing in position.
34. **Sustained release dosage forms (W. 98, 00, 05):** These are the new drug delivery systems which provide a therapeutic

blood level of drug which is attained rapidly and is maintained usually for 10 to 12 hours.

Advantages of Sustained Release Dosage Forms

1. Avoid frequent drug administration.
2. Longer duration of action.
3. Provide uniform blood concentration of drug.
4. Increase patient compliance.

Disadvantages of Sustained Release Dosage Forms

1. Not 100% efficient.
2. Adverse effects of certain drugs are difficult to control.

6 Give merits and demerits of solid dosage forms. (W. 97, 08)

☞ **Merits**

1. Unit dose system.
2. Provides stability.
3. Economical.
4. Ease of administration.
5. Rapid dissolution.
6. Sustained release dosage is possible.
7. Simplicity in production.

Demerits

1. Difficult to swallow by some children, e.g. tablet.
2. Not useful in unconscious patient.
3. Onset of action is slow.
4. Some drugs may cause GIT irritation.

7 Give merits and demerits of liquid dosage forms. (S. 99, 04)

☞ **Merits**

1. Onset of action is quick as compared to tablets and capsules.
2. Certain medicaments can only be given in liquid form, e.g. castor oil.

3. Certain drugs are to be given in suspended form to produce maximum surface area.
4. A few drugs if taken in dry form may cause pain and irritation.
5. Psychological satisfaction to a patient of something is in the bottle.

Demerits

1. Dose has to be measured.
2. Stability and preservation possess a problem.
3. Storage should be proper.
4. Possibility of breaking the containers during transport.
5. Costly dosage form than the solid dosage form.

8 **Write a note on "modern drug delivery system" or "new drug delivery system" or "novel drug delivery system" or "nonimmediate drug delivery system" or "sustained release dosage forms". (S. 07, 08; W. 02, 04)**

☞ With the advancement in pharmaceutical sciences various modern dosage forms are designed. These are:

1. Implants.
2. Films and stirps.
3. Liposome drug carriers.
4. Controlled drug delivery modules.
5. Erythrocytes.
6. Nanoparticles.
7. Prodrugs.

1. Implants

– These are sterile solid bodies placed below the skin by means of minor surgery.
– They release the drug slowly and produce prolonged drug action.

2. Films and Strips

– They are applied on affected area.
– These contain a drug which releases slowly for a specific period.

3. Liposome Drug Carriers

– Liposomes are one of the carrier systems in the body.

- The drug is enclosed in the liposomes and during its circulation the drug is delivered at the targeted site.

4. Controlled Drug Delivery Modules (CDDM)

- These are the devices prepared by embedding the drug within the polymeric matrix like polythene, cellulose, etc.
- The drug releases slowly through matrix and produces prolonged drug action.

5. Erythrocytes (RBCs)

- These are used to give controlled release of drugs.
- The life span of erythrocytes is 120 days.
- When the drug is enclosed in the erythrocytes, it diffuses out slowly from cell during its circulation and produces prolonged drug action.

6. Nanoparticles

- It is based on colloidal drug delivery system.
- The particle size of this system is 200–500 nm.
- The system consists of a drug and a carrier to deposit the drug at the target site.
- Usually naturally occurring macromolecules like human serum albumin, etc. used as a carrier.

Advantages of Novel Drug Delivery System

1. Frequency of drug administration is reduced.
2. Patient compliance is improved.
3. Better control of plasma level of drug.
4. Dose of drug is reduced.
5. Cost of therapy is reduced.

Disadvantages of Novel Drug Delivery System

1. Dose dumping may occur.
2. Dosage adjustment is difficult.
3. Termination of therapy is difficult.
4. In certain cases minor surgery is required, e.g. implants.
5. Fluctuations in *in vitro* and *in vivo* results.

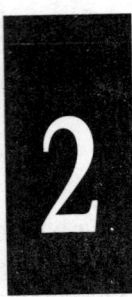

Introduction to Pharmacopoeia

1 **What is pharmacopoeia?/Define pharmacopoeia. (S. 97, 98, 02, 04, 05, 07, 08, 09; W. 00, 02)**

☞ **Pharmacopoeia**

Pharmacopoeia is the official book of standards published by respective governments containing the list of drugs, pharmaceuticals, their formulae, identification, standardisation, dose, uses, etc.

The word pharmacopoeia is derived from two Greek words:
'Pharmacon' means 'drug'
'Poeio' means 'To make'.

2 **What is object/need/purpose and scope of pharmacopoeia? (S. 08)**

☞ Pharmacopoeias are published or needed:
   (i) To ensure uniformity in composition of drug.
   (ii) To ensure purity of drug.
   (iii) To ensure potency of drug.
   (iv) To study official preparations of drugs.
   (v) To refer procedures for testing of drugs.

3 **Why "there is no world pharmacopoeia" published?**

☞ There is no single book like world pharmacopoeia because:
   (i) Pharmacopoeia is a book of standards published by respective government.

(ii) The drugs or the standards which are used in different parts of the world are different.

4 Give the list of official or standard books/pharmacopoeias published by WHO. (S. 08)

☞ 1. Indian pharmacopoeia (IP).
2. British pharmacopoeia (BP).
3. International pharmacopoeia.
4. United State pharmacopoeia (USP).
5. British pharmaceutical codex (BPC).
6. National formulary (NF).
7. Merk index.
8. European pharmacopoeia.

5 What are the contents of pharmacopoeia? Define 'monograph'.

☞ Indian pharmacopoeia contains:
(a) Monograph

(i) Main title	(vi) Description
(ii) Synonym	(vii) Solubility
(iii) Chemical formula	(viii) Standards
(iv) Category	(ix) Identification
(v) Dose	(x) Test for purity

(b) Appendices

Monograph

It means detail study of drug with reference to title, synonym, preparation, storage, category, official preparations, etc.

6 Describe the "history of Indian pharmacopoeia". (S. 97, 98, 99, 02, 03, 05; W. 98, 04)

☞ • The government of India in 1944 directed the "Drug Technical Advisory Board" to list the drugs which are not published in British pharmacopoeia.
• To that effect government of India published "Indian pharmacopoeial list" in 1946.
• In 1948, Dr BN Ghosh prepared the first edition of Indian pharmacopoeia.

- First edition of pharmacopoeia was published in 1955 and was in Latin.
- Second edition of IP was published in 1966.
- Second edition of IP was prepared under the chairmanship of Dr Mukharji and its supplements were published in 1975.
- Third edition of IP was published in 1985.
- Third edition of IP was published in two volumes namely Volume I and Volume II.
- Fourth edition was published in 1996.
- Supplements to IP 85 were published in 1989 and in 1991.

7 **Give the salient features of IP 66 (second edition).**

☞1. Titles of monograph have been changed from Latin to English.
2. Doses are expressed in metric system.
3. Solubility is expressed in parts of solvents.
4. The methods of preparation of the drug have been given immediately after the monograph.
5. New analytical techniques have been introduced.
6. The test for sterility has been modified.

8 **Give the salient features of IP 85 (third edition). (S. 99, 04, 06; W. 98, 00, 02, 05, 06, 07, 08)**

☞1. The new analytical techniques such as flamephometry, fluorometry are introduced.
2. Dissolution test has been introduced in case of certain tablets.
3. Disintegration tests for tablets have been modified.
4. Pyrogen test is also modified.
5. Some drugs have been renamed, e.g. acetyl salicylic acid: aspirin.
6. Certain drugs are omitted and some drugs are newly added.
7. Test for determination of viscosity has been modified.
8. Many new broad-spectrum antibiotics are included.
9. Microbial test limits are prescribed for certain types of oral liquids and pharmaceutical aids.
10. IUPAC system of nomenclature of organic compounds has been used.

9 Write a note on "National Formulary of India" (NF). (S. 00, 06; W. 99)

☞ National Formulary of India was published for the guidance of medical practitioners, medical students, pharmacists in hospitals and sales department.

- The first edition of National Formulary was published in 1960 by Government of India, Ministry of Health.
- The second edition of National Formulary was published in 1966, under chairmanship of Dr BB Yodh.
- The third edition of National Formulary was published in 1979 under the chairmanship of Dr Wig KL.
- In third edition of NF 342 new formulations were added and separate chapters on drug interactions, drug dependence, prescription writing were included.

10 Give the salient features of fourth edition of Indian pharmacopoeia (IP 1996). (W. 06, 07, 08)

☞ 1. It contains 1149 monographs and 123 appendices and is available in two volumes.
2. The new analytical technique like HPLC is included.
3. Some titles have been changed to include more commonly accepted names, e.g. hyoscine hydrobromide for scopolamine hydrobromide.
4. The computer generated structural formulae have been introduced.
5. The test for bacterial endotoxin (LAL test) as a more suitable substitute for the test for pyrogen has been included.
6. A number of general monographs, e.g. eyedrops, eye ointments, suppositories, pessaries, oral liquid, nasal preparations have been included.

Metrology

1 Define 'metrology'. Enlist various systems of weights and measures. (W. 96, 00, 04, 08)

☞ Metrology is the branch of science that deals with study of systems of weights and measures. There are two main systems of weights and measures followed in pharmacy:

    (i) Metric system (Decimal system)
    (ii) Imperial system (English system)
        (a) Avoirdupois
        (b) Apothecaries.

2 What do you mean by 'isotonic', paratonic', 'hypertonic', 'hypotonic' solutions?

☞ **Isotonic Solutions (S. 97, 04, 08; W. 98, 01, 05)**

The solutions having some osmotic pressure as that of plasma are known as isotonic solutions (iso-osmotic solution).

Paratonic Solutions

The solutions having different osmotic pressure as compared to plasma are called paratonic solutions.

Hypotonic Solutions (S. 97; W. 98, 01)

The solutions having lower osmotic pressure than the plasma are called hypotonic solutions.

Hypertonic Solutions (S. 97; W. 98, 01)

The solutions having osmotic pressure higher than plasma are called hypertonic solutions.

3 What is effect of injecting hypotonic and hypertonic solutions in bloodstream? (S. 05; W. 03, 04, 08)

☞ 1. If hypotonic solution is administered parenterally, endo-osmosis will occur resulting in haemolysis of RBCs (breakdown of RBCs).

2. If hypertonic solution is administered parenterally, exo-osmosis will occur, i.e. fluid from RBCs diffuses outside and cells shrink (crenulation occurs).

Thus hypotonic solutions are more dangerous than hypertonic solutions, if administered parenterally.

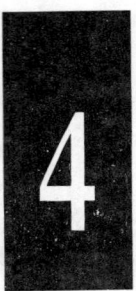

Packaging of Pharmaceuticals

1 Define container. Name the materials used for container. (S. 97, 98, 03; W. 96, 98, 02)

☞ **Container**

It is the device that holds the drug and may or may not contact with drug.
  • Materials used: Glass, plastic, metals, paper, board, etc.

2 Define closure. Name the materials used for closure. (S. 97, 98, 03; W. 98, 01, 02)

☞ **Closure**

It is the device by means of which container can be closed and opened.
  • Materials used: Glass, plastic, rubber, metal, cork.

3 Define 'package' and 'packaging'.

☞ **Package (S. 99)**

A package consists of:
  1. A container which holds the product.
  2. Closure which seals the container.
  3. The carton (outer cover) which gives protection.
  4. The box in which multiples of product are packed.

Packaging (S. 99)

It is the science and technology which deals with study of materials and methods used to pack the product and also provide the knowledge of the machinery used for packing the product.

4 What are the ideal qualities of a container? (S. 07, 08; W. 04, 07)

☞• It should hold the product without loss.
 • It should protect the drug from air, moisture, light, dust, etc.
 • It should be neutral.
 • It should not wear and tear during normal handling.
 • It should pour the drug properly.
 • It should not be affected by temperature and pressure.
 • It should not break during handling and transportation.
 • It should be nontoxic.
 • It sholuld be attractive in size and shape.

5 What are various types of containers? (S. 98, 00, 01, 05; W. 97, 98, 01, 06, 08)

☞ According to protection provided by the container, they are classified as:

1. **Well closed container:** It protects the products from the loss during transportation, handling, storage, etc.

2. **Tightly closed container:** It protects the drug from contamination due to solids or liquids and also prevents loss due to evaporation.

3. **Airtight container/hermatically sealed container:** It prevents the entry of air inside the container during handling, distribution, storage, etc. For example, required for injectables.

4. **Light resistant container:** It protects the product from harmful effects of light. Usually amber-coloured glass is used. It is useful for photosensitive durgs.

5. **Tamper evident/tamperproof container:** It is fitted with device of mechanism that proves; where container has been opened.

6. **Single dose container:** It contains only single dose of the drug. It is usually used for injectables, e.g. ampoules.

7. **Multidose container:** It contains more than one dose of a drug, e.g. vials.

8. **Aerosol container:** It is used to hold aerosol products.

6 **Give merits and demerits of glass. Why is glass used as a packaging material? (S. 99; W. 96, 03, 05)**

☞ **Glass**

Merits

1. It is transparent.
2. It is available in various shapes and sizes.
3. Not affected by temperature and pressure during sterilization.
4. It is neutral.
5. It is economical.
6. Light sensitive drugs can be stored in amber-coloured glass.
7. It is impermeable.
8. It has good protection power.
9. It does not deteriorate with age.

Demerits

1. Easily breakable.
2. Some glasses relese alkali.
3. Bulk package should be labelled as: "Glass: Handle with care."
4. Chances of flake formation.

7 **Discuss plastic as a material for packaging. (S. 99, 04, 05; W. 00, 07)**

☞ **Plastic**

Merits

1. They are light in weight and can be handled easily.
2. Available in various shapes and sizes.
3. They are unbreakable.
4. They can be transported easily.
5. Resistant to inorganic chemicals.
6. Bad conductor of heat.
7. Good protection power.
8. They have sufficient mechanical strength.

Demerits

1. They may absorb the product.
2. Leaching problem.
3. Discolouration of the product.
4. Some plastics are permeable to gases, moisture, etc.

8 **What is closure? Give its importance. Explain types of closure. (S. 06; W. 00, 02, 06)**

☞ **Closure**

It is the device by means of which container can be closed and opened.

Advantages/Importance

1. To protect the drug from air, dust, moisture, etc.
2. To prevent loss of preparation during handling.

Types of Closures

1. **Plug type:** It is fitted into the neck of the container, e.g. cork, rubber, glass stopper.

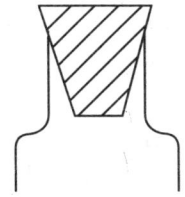

2. **Crown cap:** It is used for packing of beverage bottles, e.g. metals.

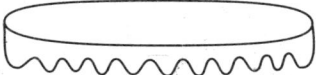

3. **Push-fit type:** It is simple slide fit over the neck of the container, e.g. plastic caps.

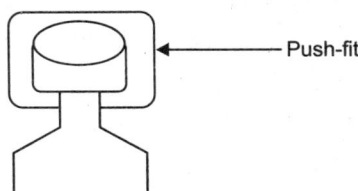

Push-fit

4. **Screw-cap:** It is very commonly used.

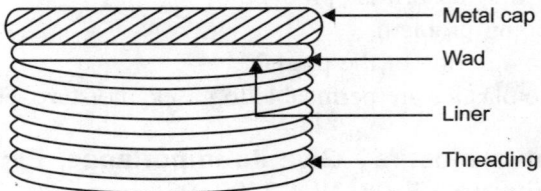

Metal cap
Wad
Liner
Threading

9 What are the ideal requirements of rubber closure? (S. 04, 06, 07, 08)

☞ An ideal rubber closure must possess following properties:
1. It should be soft.
2. It should be quite elastic.
3. It should not absorb medicament.
4. It should withstand temperature and pressure of autoclave.
5. It should be compatible with product.
6. It should comply with pharmacopoeial standards.
7. It should be impermeable to moisture and air.
8. It should not release any substance in the product.

10 What are the various tests used for rubber closure?/ (Official tests/evaluation tests/pharmacopoeial tests.) (S. 96, 08; W. 96, 97, 01)

☞ 1. **Test for penetrability:** Rubber should have sufficient softners to penetrate the needle through it. Thus hardness of the rubber closure is tested.
2. **Extractive test:** The rubber should not extract out the materials present in it beyond the prescribed limit.
3. **Fragmentation test:** Fragmentation of rubber due to penetration of hypodermic needle should be within the range.
4. **Permeability test:** It is performed to test permeability of the rubber to the water vapours.
5. **Compatibility test:** It is performed to ensure that there is no interaction between the rubber closure and the contents of product.

11 What is tamperproof/evident (resistant) container?

☞ **Tamperproof Container**

It is one having an indicator barrier to entry, which, if broken or missing, can provide visible evidence to the buyer that the product has been tampered or opened.

Tamper evident packaging are classified as:
1. Strip packaging
2. Blister packaging
3. Film wrappers
4. Bottle seal
5. Breakable caps
6. Sealed tubes
7. Sealed cartons
8. Bubble packs
9. Foil paper or plastic pouches
10. Aerosol.

12 Define aerosol. What are the types of aerosols? (S. 96, 97, 02, 03; W. 97, 98)

☞ **Aerosol**

It is a dispersed system in which very fine solid particles or liquid droplets are dispersed in the gas, which act as a continuous phase.

These are also called pressurized dosage forms.

Types of Aerosol (Classification of Aerosols)

1. **Space aerosol/spray:** It contains finely divided particles having particle size 50 μ, e.g. insecticide spray.
2. **Surface coat aerosol/spray:** It contains dispersed particles having particle size 200 μ, e.g. hair spray, personal deodoriser.
3. **Foam aerosol/spray:** In this type the product comes out in the form of foam from the container, e.g. shaving cream.

13 Give advantages and disadvantages of aerosol. (S. 97, 02, 03; W. 98, 04, 07, 08)

☞ **Advantages**

1. It is directly applied on affected area.
2. It minimises discomfort caused by manual applied.

3. Ease of application.
4. Absence of air prevents oxidation of product.
5. The hydrolysis of medicament can be prevented.
6. Drug can be given by oral inhalation.
7. The sterility of product can be maintained.
8. Manual contact with medicament can be avoided.

Disadvantages

1. Aerosols are costly preparations.
2. Some of the propellants are very costly.
3. Some propellants irritate the injured parts.
4. Some propellants produce toxic effects.
5. These should be kept away from the children.
6. Many difficulties are faced in aerosol formulation.

14 Write a note on formulation of aerosol. What are the types of aerosol systems? (S. 09; W. 03)

☞ Formulation of Aerosol

Aerosol contains following additives:

(a) **Propellant:** It is used to develop pressure inside the container.
   - For this purpose compressed gases like CO_2, N_2 liquified gases like ethane, methane can be used as a propellant.
   - For pharmaceutical aerosol propellants used are:
     1. Trichloro-fluoro methane
     2. Dichloro-fluoroethane
     3. Dichloro-tetra-fluoroethane
     4. Difluoro-ethane.

(b) **Medicament:** It may be solid or liquid and may be soluble or insoluble in the propellant.

(c) **Other additives:** It includes flavouring agent, antioxidant, solvents, surface active agents.

Types of Aerosol Systems

1. Two-Phase System

In this system the medicament (solid/liquid) is soluble in the propellant or solid is insoluble in the propellant and is dispersed in the propellant. Thus aerosol system has two phases, one is liquid while other is gaseous. Hence called two-phase aerosol system.

2. Three-Phase Aerosol System

In this system the medicament is insoluble in propellant and it is dissolved in the liquid which is immiscible with the propellant.

Thus, there are three phases namely:

1. Propellant
2. Immiscible liquid
3. Gaseous phase.

Thus, it is known as three-phase aerosol system.

15 **Give the construction of aerosol container. (S. 96, 97, 02, 03, 07; W. 97, 98, 04, 07, 08)**

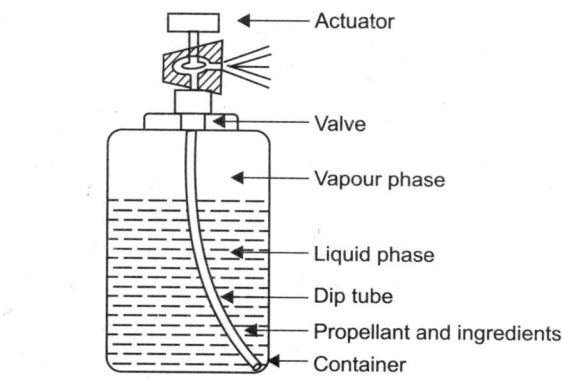

Aerosol container can be divided into four parts:

Container

It is constructed from metals, glass or plastic.

- The metals used are aluminium, stainless steel, etc.
- The container shall be such that it can withstand high pressure.

Valves

The valves should be easily opened and closed.

It should spray the content in desired form.

Three types of valves are used nowadays:

1. Continuous spray valve: This valve expels medicament continuously as long as actuator is pressed.
2. Metering valve: This valve expels a metered dose when actuator is pressed.
3. Foam value: This valve expels the contents in the form of foam when actuator is pressed.

Actuator

It is fitted on the valve stem.

It helps in the easy opening and closing of the valve.

Dip Tube

It is made up of polythene or polypropylene.

It is used for two purposes:

1. It conveys the liquid from the bottom of the container to the valve at the top.
2. It prevents the propellant to come out without dispensing the contents of the package.

16 What are pharmaceutical applications of aerosol packages?

☞1. They are used for spray bandages and for application of drugs for topical use.
2. They are used for administration of drugs into various body cavities.
3. They are used for administration of drugs such as local anaesthetics, local antiseptics, local analgesics, etc.
4. They are used to spray cosmetic preparations such as perfumes.
5. They are used to spray disinfectants, deodorizers and air sanitizers.

17 Write a note on flexible packages. (S. 99)

☞• These are used for packing of all types of products like solids, semisolids and also liquids.
• The concept of unit dose packaging in making flexible packages is more popular.
• The materials used for flexible packages are paper, plastic film, aluminium foil or combination of these two.
• Paper is widely used for drug and cosmetic packaging due to its light weight, enough strength, economy and convenience.
• Coated and laminated papers are more advantageous.
• Heat seal aluminium foil is most suitable for packaging of pharmaceutical products.
• Flexible packages are useful for unit containers.
• Strip-packed tablets and capsules are very popular.
• Cellophane is a material of choice for flexible packaging.

Size Reduction

1 Define size reduction. Give importance/significance of size reduction in pharmacy. (S. 96, 97, 00, 05; W. 97, 98, 00, 01)

☞ **Size Reduction**

Size reduction is the process of reducing drugs into smaller pieces, coarse particles or fine powder.

Importance/Significance of Size Reduction

1. It increases rate of dissolution of drug.
2. It increases rate of absorption of drug.
3. It helps in extraction process.
4. It increases stability of the preparation.
5. It increases solubility of the drug.
6. It gives proper consistency to the preparation.
7. It increases uniformity and elegance of the preparation.
8. It helps in drying of various drugs.
9. It provides uniform mixing of the particles.
10. It helps in size separation.

2 Discuss various factors affecting size reduction. (S. 03, 04, 05, 08, 09; W. 98, 03, 07)

☞(a) **Hardness:** It is easy to break soft material than hard material.
  (b) **Toughness:** Fibrous drugs or having higher moisture content are generally soft but tough. Thus they produce difficulties in size reduction.

(c) **Stickness:** Drugs like gums, resins are sticky and may adhere to the grinding surfaces. Thus stickness creates difficulties in size reduction.

(d) **Moisture content:** The presence of moisture in the material affects hardness, toughness and stickness. Thus drugs containing high moisture content are difficult to reduce their size.

(e) **Material structure:** Vegetative drugs produce fibrous particles while minerals produce flakes.

(f) **Softening temperature:** During size reduction heat is generated, so some drugs may melt during size reduction.

(g) **Physiological effect:** During size reduction dust is produced which is dangerous to workers.

(h) **Ratio of feed size and product size:** If feed size is large the coarse particles are obtained.

(i) **Purity required:** Due to wear and tear of the parts of machine, product may contaminate.

3 What are the principles/mechanism involved in size reduction methods? (S. 00, 01, 06, 07, 09; W. 04)

☞(a) **Cutting:** The material is cut into small pieces by a sharp blade, or knife, e.g. cutter mill.

(b) **Compression:** The material is crushed by application of pressure, e.g. roller mill.

(c) **Impact:** In this case material is hit by an object moving at high speed and material breaks into smaller pieces, e.g. hammer mill, disintegrator.

(d) **Attrition:** In this case mechanical pressure is applied on the material in two moving surfaces, resulting in shear forces which break the particles, e.g. roller mill.

(e) **Combined impact and attrition:** In this case both impact and attrition are involved to get better results, e.g. ball mill, fluid energy mill.

4 Write a note on hammer mill. (S. 03; W. 97, 05)

☞ It is based on the principle of impact.
   • **Construction:** It consists of strong metal casing enclosing central shaft to which many hammers are fixed. At the lower

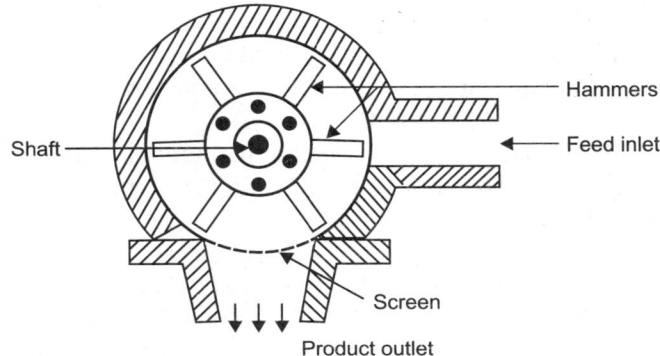

side there is a screen through which powder passes. There is a feed inlet and product outlet.

- **Working:** During operation, central shaft rotates with high speed. The hammers bite the material entering from feed inlet and powdered material is collected through the outlet.
- **Advantage:** It is used for producing intermediate grade of powder.
- **Disadvantage:** Due to high speed heat is generated and therefore, it is not suitable for heat-sensitive materials.

5 Write a note on disintegrator. (S. 01, 03, 04; W. 98)

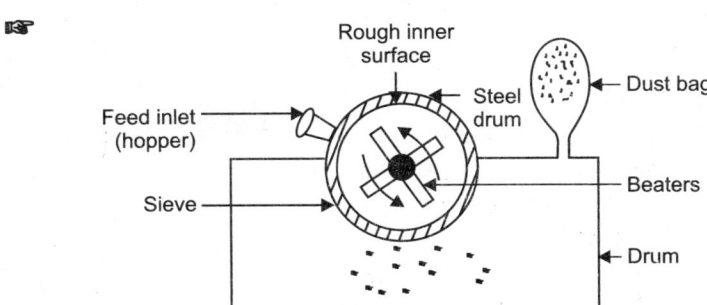

- **Principle of working:** Impact.
- **Construction:** It consists of steel drum having shaft in the centre. Shaft contains disc on which four beaters are fixed. The shaft rotates with the speed of 500–700 revolutions per minute. The upper inner surface of the drum is rough and lower part of

the drum has sieve. The material entering through hopper is broken into small particles by impact of beaters. The grinding also occurs because of striking of particles on the rough upper surface of the steel drum.

- **Dust bag:** Dust bag is attached to the outlet through which air is allowed to pass and helps to retain the dust carried by air.
- **Advantages**
    (i) Useful for grinding of vegetable drugs.
    (ii) Useful for powdering of hard material.
    (iii) Useful for mixing of different powdered ingredients.
- **Disadvantage:** Possibility of jamming of beaters if large pieces of material enter in it.

6 **Write a note on fluid energy mill. (S. 96, 99, 00, 01, 02, 03, 05, 08; W. 99, 01, 04, 06, 07, 08)**

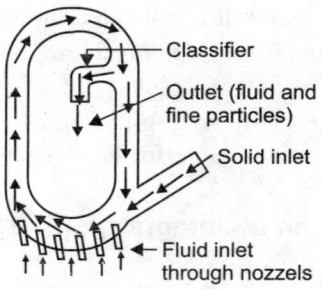

- **Principle:** Combined impact and attrition.
- **Construction:**
    (i) It consists of a loop of pipe having diameter 20 mm to 200 mm and height about 2 metres.
    (ii) It has solid inlet and fluid inlet.
    (iii) At the top there is a classifier which allows fluid to pass but prevents particles to pass until they become sufficiently fine.
- **Working:** The fluid is introduced under very high pressure through the nozzles. The solids to be powdered are introduced into the air stream through solid inlet. Due to high degree of turbulance, **impact and attrition** occur between the particles resulting in size reduction.

The fine particles are collected through classifier.

- **Advantages:**
  - (i) Used to obtain particles in μ size.
  - (ii) Particle size can be controlled by using classifier.
  - (iii) No wear and tear of mill.
  - (iv) Suitable for heat sensitive materials.
- **Disadvantages:**
  - (i) Premilling of material is required.
  - (ii) Controlled supply of feed is required.

7 Write a note on ball mill. (S. 98, 04; W. 96, 01, 02, 04, 07)

☞• **Principle:** Combined impact and attrition.

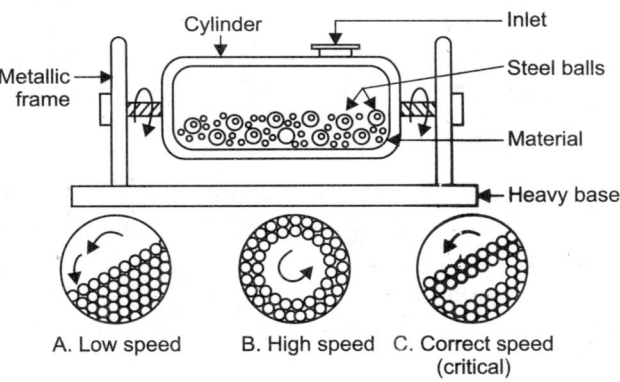

A. Low speed   B. High speed   C. Correct speed (critical)

Figure 'A': At low speed, there is very negligible size reduction.
Figure 'B': At very high speed, balls will thrown out due to centrifugal force. Hence no grinding will occur.
Figure 'C': At critical speed, the balls fall on the material and maximum size reduction will occur.

- **Construction:**
  - (i) It consists of hollow cylinder fixed on metallic frame.
  - (ii) It contains steel heavy balls about 2–5 cm in diameter.
  - (iii) Sometimes cylinders are lined with rubber.
  - (iv) The cylinder revolves longitudinally.
- **Working:**
  - (i) The drug is placed into the cylinder and lid is closed.
  - (ii) The cylinder rotates longitudinally.
  - (iii) The speed of rotation is very important.

- **Advantages:**
    - (i) It can produce very fine powder.
    - (ii) It can be used for continuous operation, if sieve is attached to mill.
    - (iii) Toxic materials can be reduced, as it is closed to mill.
    - (iv) It is useful in large scale.
    - (v) It is capable of grinding wide variety of materials of different degree of hardness.
- **Disadvantages:**
    - (i) It is very noisy machine.
    - (ii) Wear and tear of balls may contaminate the product.
    - (iii) Not suitable for sticky materials.
    - (iv) Regular maintenance is required.

8 **What is levigation? Describe the role of levigating agents with examples. (S. 03, 07; W. 01, 02)**

☞ **Levigation**

Levigation is the process of wet grinding in which the material is converted into fine powder with the help of insoluble liquid known as levigating agent.

- After levigation the paste is obtained which consists of large proportion of the fine particles along with a small proportion of coarse particles.
- Levigation method can be done by using morter and pastle and by using tile and spatula.
- This method is used for the preparation of ointments, suspension, etc.
- Commercially, levigation is used for the preparation of light kaolin, chalk, calamine.

Role of Levigating Agents

The insoluble liquids used for levigation are called levigating agents, e.g. water, liquid paraffin, glycerin. Levigating agents prevent the feeling of grittiness in the preparation due to solid drug present.

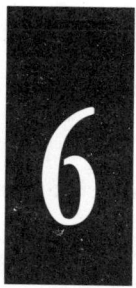

Size Separation

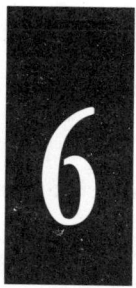 **Define size separation. What are various official standards for powders/grading of solids (Classify powders)? (S. 97, 99, 00, 03, 04, 05, 07, 08, 09; W. 97, 99, 04, 05, 07, 08)**

☞ **Size Separation**

It is a technique used to separate the particles of specified size.

Official Standards for Powders

Grade of powder	Sieve through which all particles must pass	Sieve through which only 40% of particles pass
1. Coarse powder	10	44
2. Moderately coarse powder	22	60
3. Moderately fine powder	44	85
4. Fine powder	85	–
5. Very fine powder	120	–

Definitions

1. **Coarse powder:** It is the powder of which all the particles pass through sieve no. 10 and not more than 40% pass through sieve no. 44.
2. **Moderately coarse powder:** It is the powder of which all the particles pass through sieve no. 22 and not more than 40% pass through sieve no. 60.

3. **Moderately fine powder:** It is the powder of which all the particles pass through sieve no. 44 and not more than 40% pass through sieve no. 85.
4. **Fine powder:** It is the powder of which all the particles pass through sieve no. 85.
5. **Very fine powder:** It is the powder of which all the particles pass through sieve no. 120.

2 **Define the terms 'sieve no.', sieve no. 10'. (S. 04, 09; W. 04, 08)**

☞(a) **Sieve no.:** It means number of meshes in a length of 2.54 cm (1 inch) in each transverse direction parallel to the wire.
  (b) **Sieve no. 10:** It means 10 number of meshes in a length of 2.54 cm (1 inch) in each transverse direction parallel to the wire.

3 **Name various methods used for size separation. (S. 05; W. 06)**

☞ 1. Sieving/screening.
  2. Cyclone separator.
  3. Air separator.
  4. Elutriation/sedimentation.
  5. Centrifugal classification.

4 **Give the construction and working of cyclone separator. (S. 96, 98, 01, 03, 06, 08, 09; W. 96, 97, 99, 02, 04, 05, 07)**

☞

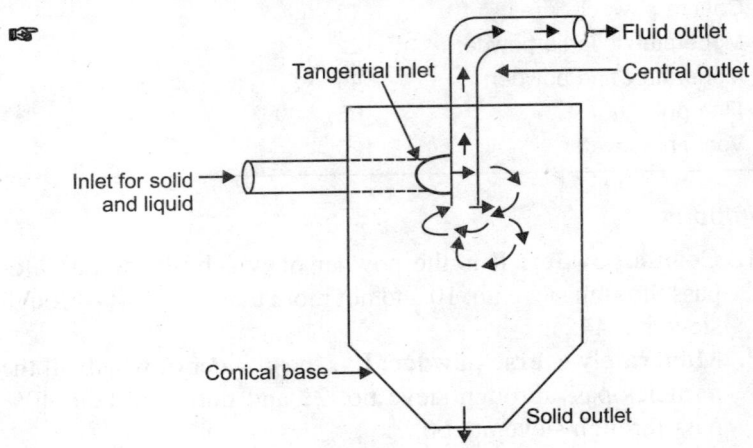

Principle

In cyclone separator centrifugal force is used to separate solids from the fluid. Separation depends not only on the particle size but also on the density of particles.

Construction

In consists of cylindrical vessel with conical base.
- It has fluid outlet at the top and solid outlet at bottom.
- There is a tangential inlet through which suspension is passed.

Working

The suspension of solid in gas or liquid is introduced under very high velocity into the vessel so that rotatory movements take place within the vessel. Due to centrifugal force the particles having high density are thrown towards the wall and are collected through conical base. The fine particles are collected along with the fluid.

5 ▎ What is elutriation? Explain. (S. 06, 09; W. 98)

☞

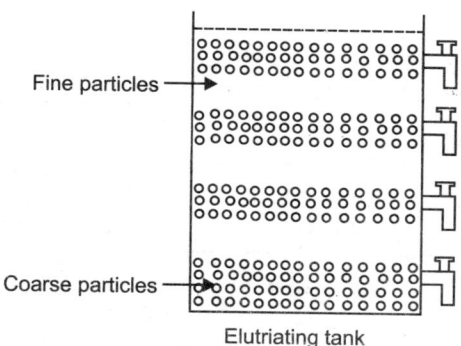

Fine particles →

Coarse particles →

Elutriating tank

Elutriation

Elutriation is the process of size separation of the particles depending on their particle size and density.

Principle

In the elutriation method size separation is based on the principle of low density of fine particles and high density of coarse particles.

Elutriating tank is used to separate the fine particles from the coarse particles from the powder or paste obtained after levigation. The powder or paste is mixed with the water in the elutriating tank and liquid is stirred and allowed to settle down. Depending upon the density of particles, they will either settle or remain suspended in water at different levels. The sample is withdrawn at different heights through the outlets and then they are dried to get powder with various size fractions.

6 **Describe sedimentation method of size separation. OR Explain sedimentation tanks. (S. 01, 02; W. 08)**

☞ **Sedimentation**

It is the process in which insoluble particles settle down due to the gravity depending upon their densities.

- Sedimentation is one of the methods used in size separation.
- Sedimentation tanks are used for this process.
- Sedimentation tanks

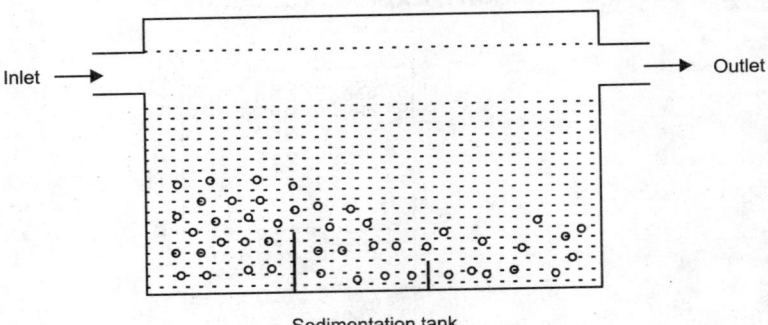

Sedimentation tank

- The sedimentation tank works on the following principle:
  - Insoluble particles settle down due to the gravity.
  - The rate of sedimentation of particles is governed by Stokes law equation.

$$V \propto \frac{2r^2(e-e_0)p}{gn}$$

where, r = Radius of the particle
p = Density of the particle
n = Viscosity of the medium.

- Sedimentation tanks are used for large scale fluid classification of solids. In this, suspension of solids in a fluid is placed in a tank. The suspension is allowed to stand for some time. The supernatant is removed and the thickened suspension is collected. The suspension may be collected at different levels giving different fractions. The suspension collected successively will then contain finer particles.
- Sometimes continuous sedimentation process may be employed for size separation.
- In this case slurry enters at one end. The particles in the slurry are acted upon by a force having a horizontal and vertical component. The horizontal component is due to flow of fluid that carries the particles in forward directions, whereas the vertical component due to gravity causes the particles to move downwards to the bottom of the tank. Thus, the coarsest particles settle near the inlet, moderately coarse at middle and fine near outlet, very fine particles may get flown out with liquid itself.

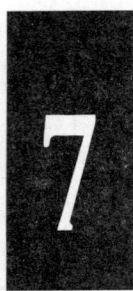

Mixing and Homogenisation

1 **What is mixing? Give the objectives of mixing. (S. 98, 02, 07, 09; W. 97, 02)**

☞ **Mixing**

Mixing is a unit operation in which two or more substances are combined together in such a way that each particle of material looks similar to particles of other material.

Objectives of Mixing

1. To form a uniform mixture.
2. To promote chemical reaction to get uniform product.
3. It helps in formation of suspension or paste.
4. It helps in mixing of water and oil, e.g. emulsion.

2 **Give the types of mixing on mixtures and their stability. (S. 96, 07; W. 96, 98, 02)**

☞ There are three types of mixtures:

1. Positive mixtures: When two or more miscible liquids are mixed together or solid is dissolved in water. Such types of mixtures are called positive mixtures.

They are irreversible and stable in nature, e.g. solutions.

2. Negative mixtures: When two immiscible liquids are mixed with water, the mixture is called negative mixture. It is reversible mixture and requires high degree of mixing of materials, e.g. emulsion.

3. **Neutral mixtures:** It is neutral in behaviour. The substances do not have tendency to mix but once they are mixed they do not separate after mixing, e.g. ointment, paste, creams.

3 **What are the mechanisms of mixing? (S. 97, 98, 99, 03, 08; W. 98, 04, 06)**

☞(a) **Convective mixing:** It means transfer of group of particles from one location to another and it is carried out by means of blades or paddles.

(b) **Shear mixing:** In this case mixing of powders takes place due to shear force.

(c) **Diffusion mixing:** It occurs due to the random motion of particles within the powdered bed which causes change in position of particles relative to each other. It is carried out by stirring.

4 **Explain factors affecting powder mixing (solid mixing). (S. 97, 98, 99, 03; W. 98)**

☞(a) **Particle size:** It is easy to mix the powders having approximately same particle size.

(b) **Particle shape:** For uniform mixing ideal particle shape should be spherical.

(c) **Density of material:** It is difficult to mix the powders having different densities.

(d) **Particle attraction:** Some particles exert attractive forces due to electrostatic charges on them.

(e) **Proportion of materials:** The materials to be mixed should be in the proportionate quantities and if they are not, they are mixed in the ascending order of their weight.

5 **Name the equipment used for mixing of solids, semisolids and liquids.**

☞

Type	Equipment used
1. Mixing of solids/ powders	Tumbler mixer, agitated powder mixer, double cone blender, air mixer
2. Mixing of semisolids	Triple roller mill, agitated mixer, sigma blade mixer
3. Mixing of liquids	Propeller mixer, turbine mixer, paddle mixer

6 Write a note on double cone blender (mixer). (S. 03; W. 96, 97, 00)

☞ It is also known as twin shell blender.

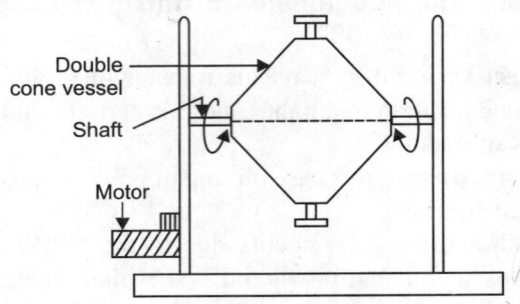

Mechanism

Diffusion mixing.

Construction

It consists of two cone-shaped vessels fixed base to base and mounted in shaft. It is made up of stainless steel. The shaft is fixed and cone-shaped vessel revolves at optimum speed. The apparatus is connected to an electric driven motor.

Working

The solids to be mixed are taken in the conical shape vessel. Due to rotation, material moves to top and falls down at the bottom. Mixing takes place by tumbling of vessel and by diffusion.

Applications

(a) Used for mixing of powders to be filled in capsules.
(b) Mixing and lubrication of granules.

7 Write a note on "triple roller mill". (S. 96, 06, 07; W. 97, 98, 99, 04, 08)

☞ It is used for mixing of semisolids.

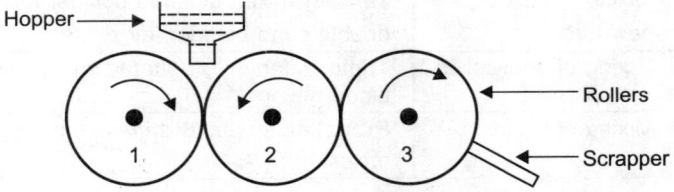

Mechanism

Shear mixing.

Construction

1. It consists of three rollers which are arranged in such a way that they come very close to each other.
2. The rollers are rotated at different rates of speed.
3. Hopper is located above the 1st and 2nd roller.
4. Scrapper helps to remove the material from the roller.

Working

1. As shown in figure, material is supplied in between roller 1 and 2 and it gets reduced.
2. The gap between 2 and 3 is usually less than 1 and 2 roller.
3. A scrapper is arranged to the 3rd roller which removes the fixed material.

Application

It is used for grinding as well as for mixing of solid powders with the ointment base.

8 Define homogenisation. Describe silversion mixer homogeniser. (S. 99, 02, 06; W. 97, 02, 03, 04, 06)

☞ Homogenisation

It in refers to mixing of biphasic liquid systems in which product with uniform quality and consistency is produced.

- It is useful for preparation of fine suspension and emulsions.
- It is carried out in the apparatus known as homogenizer.

Silversion Mixer Homogeniser

Construction

1. It consists of emulsifier head, covered with stainless steel sieve.
2. Emulsifier head consists of blades attached to the shaft and rotates at high speed.
3. Electric motor is fitted at the top.

Working

1. Emulsifier head is placed in the vessel containing immiscible liquids.

2. When motor is started the liquid gets sucked through fine holes and is reduced with the help of rotating blades.

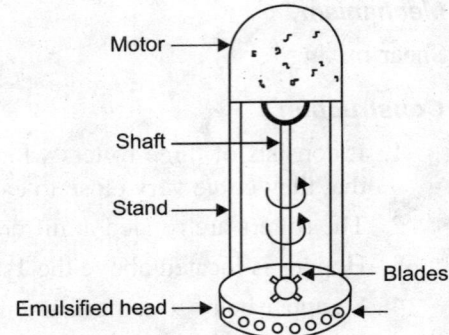

8

Filtration and Clarification

1 **Define filtration and clarification. (S. 99, 01, 04; W. 96, 06, 07)**

☞ **Filtration**

It is the process in which insoluble solids are removed from the liquid, by passing through a porous medium in which solids are retained and liquid is allowed to pass.

Clarification

It is the process of removal of relatively small amounts of suspended solids (> 0.15%) present in the liquid without using filter.

2 **Define the terms: (S. 04, 09; W. 96)**

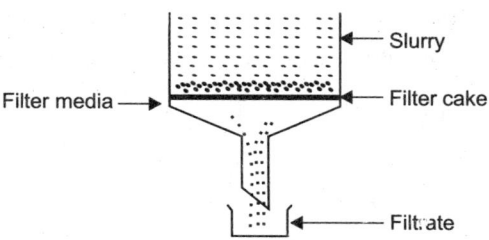

(a) **Slurry:** It is the suspension of solids to be filtered.
(b) **Filter medium:** It is the porous medium which retains the solids and allow the liquid to pass.

(c) **Filter cake:** The deposited layer of solids on the filter medium is called filter cake.

(d) **Filtrate:** It is the clear liquid passing through the filter.

(e) **Colation/straining:** When object of filtration is to remove large visible particles by using a coarse filtering medium like muslin cloth, glass wool, cotton wool, etc. Such process is known as straining/colation.

3 Distinguish between filtration and clarification. (S. 06; W. 98, 99, 04)

☞

Filtration	Clarification
(i) Filter medium is required	Filter medium is not required
(ii) Useful for removal of large amount of solids	Useful for removal of small amount of solids
(iii) Any percentage of solids can be removed	Only less than 0.15% of solids can be removed
(iv) Bacterial filtration can be possible	Cannot be used for bacterial filtration
(v) Useful for filtration of injection, eyedrops	Useful for filtration of syrups, honey
(vi) Equipment used: Filter press, candle filter, filter leaf	Equipment used: Metafilter, stream line filter

4 Describe theory of filtration/Darcy's law of filtration. (S. 97, 99; W. 02, 03, 04)

☞ The theory of filtration gives the idea about rate of filtration and is explained by Darcy.

Scientist Darcy studied the factors affecting rate of filtration and equation derived is known as Darcy's law.

Darcy's Law

$$V = \frac{KA\Delta P}{\eta l}$$

where, V = Rate of filtration

A = Area of filter bed

K = Permeability coefficient

ΔP = Pressure difference above liquid and below filter medium

η = Viscosity of liquid (slurry)

l = Thickness of filter cake.

Thus,

(i) Increase in pressure above the liquid causes increase in rate of filtration.

(ii) An increase in area increases rate of filtration.

(iii) Increase in viscosity decreases rate of filtration.

(iv) Increase is thickness of cake decreases rate of filtration.

(v) Increase in area of filter bed increases rate of filtration.

5 **Explain various factors affecting rate of filtration. (S. 04, 07, 08; W. 06)**

☞ **(a) Surface area of filter bed:** The increase in surface area of the filter bed increases the rate of filtration.

(b) Viscosity of slurry: The rate of filtration is inversely proportional to viscosity of liquid. Thus increase in viscosity decreases filtration.

(c) Thickness of cake: If thickness of filter cake is more then rate of filtration is decreased.

(d) Temperature: Increase in temperature decreases viscosity of a liquid, thus increases rate of filtration.

(e) Pressure difference: If pressure above the liquid is more than the pressure below liquid then rate of filtration is more.

(f) Particle size: Rate of filtration is directly proportional to the size of particles to be filtered. Smaller particles will block the filter media and form a cake, thus decrease rate of filtration.

6 **Define filter media. Give the ideal properties of filter media. (S. 97, 98, 00, 01, 07, 08; W. 97, 03, 05, 07)**

☞ **Filter Media**

It is the porous medium which retains the solids and allows the liquid to pass.

A good filter medium should possess following properties:

1. It should not absorb the liquid to be filtered.

2. It should have smooth surface.

3. It should be chemically inert.

4. It should have good mechanical strength.

5. It should be resistant to corrosive action of liquid.
6. It should allow free flow of liquid.
7. It should be economical.
8. It should be reusable.

7 Explain various filter medias used in pharmacy. (W. 08)

☞ (a) **Filter paper:** It is a commonly used filter medium. The filter papers are also of coarse, medium and fine pore size.
  (b) **Cotton wool:** It is used for filtering of moderately coarse particles.
  (c) **Glass wool:** It consists of fine fibres of glass which resist corrosive liquids. Hence used for filtration of strong acids and alkalies.
  (d) **Asbestos:** It is also useful for filtration of acids and alkalies.
  (e) **Fine muslin cloth:** It is used for separation of coarse particles.
  (f) **Filter cloth:** It may be both synthetic or cotton and is used for large scale filtration.
  (g) **Membrane filter:** It is made up of cellulose derivatives and used for filtration of injections, eyedrops, etc.
  (h) **Sintered glass filter:** It is made up of borosilicate glass and is used for sterile filtration.

8 Write a note on "filter aids". (S. 97, 99, 03, 06, 07; W. 99, 00, 01)

☞ **Filter Aids**

The substances which reduce the resistance to filtration and increase rate of filtration are called filter aid, e.g. talc, bentonite, kaolin, activated charcoal, diatomite, kiesel guhr.

Ideal Qualities of Filter Aids
1. It should remain suspended in the liquid.
2. It should be free from impurities.
3. It should be chemically inert and insoluble.
4. It should form porous cake.
5. It should have low specific gravity.

9 Name various equipment used for filtration.

☞ (i) Filter press.
  (ii) Filter leaf.

(iii) Filter candles.
(iv) Metafilters.
 (v) Membrane filters.
(vi) Sintered glass filters.

10 **Name the filtering devices used for sterile filtration (bacteria-proof filtration). (W. 02)**

☞   (i) Membrane filter.
   (ii) Sintered glass filter.
  (iii) Seitz filter.
  (iv) Edge filter.
   (v) Candle filter.

11 **Write a note on sintered glass filter. (S. 02; W. 01, 03, 04)**

☞ **Sintered Glass Filter**

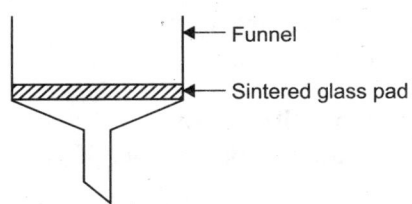

- It is made from borosilicate glass.
- The glass is powdered and sifted to produce uniform particles.
- These are heated and moulded or fused together to form a disc.
- These discs are then fitted into a suitable funnel.
- They are available in different pore sizes.
- They are graded as:

Grade 1	Pore size	90–150 μ
Grade 2	Pore size	40–90 μ
Grade 3	Pore size	15–40 μ
Grade 4	Pore size	5–15 μ
Grade 5	Pore size	up to 2 μ

Applications

1. It is useful for filtration of liquids like parenterals, corrosive liquids, oxidising agents.
2. Sintered glass filters with finest porosity are used for bacterial filtration.

12 Write a note on "membrane filter". (S. 07)

☞ These are used for ultrafiltration. These are made up of cellulose acetate, nylon or PVC as thin and flat membrane. Pore size is 400 to 500 millions per cm^2 of the filter paper. It is available in pore size of 8μ to 0.22 μ. Hence called as ultrafilter. For sterile filtration 0.22 μ to 0.45 μ pore size is used. It may get clogged therefore, prefiltration is required.

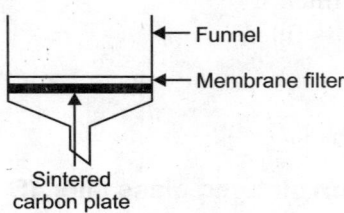

Applications

It is used for filtration and sterilisation of pharmaceutical products like eyedrops, injections, solutions, hormones, and vitamins.

13 Write a note on filter press (plate and frame filter press). (S. 98, 02, 03, 05, 09; W. 98, 99, 05, 08)

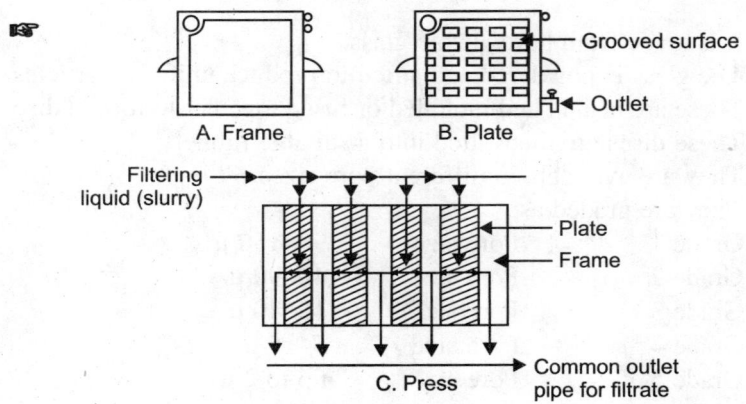

Construction

1. The filter press consists of plates and frames.
2. The frame is open and it has inlet for slurry.
3. Plate has a grooved surface which gives support to filter cloth.

4. The plate has outlet for the filtrate.
5. The plate and frame are made up of stainless steel, bronze, etc.
6. The plates and frames are placed alternately.
7. A filter cloth is positioned over each plate.
8. The whole assembly is then fitted to the outer frame of the press.
9. The outlet of each plate is connected to the common outlet pipe.

Working

As shown in Fig. (C), the slurry enters the frame under pressure from the feed channel. The filtrate passes though filter cloth on the surface of the plate. The filtrate is collected in the plate from where it is collected through common outlet pipe. The cake gets deposited in the frames. After removing cake operation may be again continued.

Advantages

1. It provides large surface area.
2. Simple in construction.
3. High filtration pressure can be used.
4. Low maintenance cost.
5. The filtering media can be used repeatedly.
6. Efficient washing of cake is possible.

Disadvantages

1. Wear of cloth is high.
2. It is not continuous process.
3. Labour cost required is more.
4. Liquid containing less than 5% solids are only filtered by this equipment.

14 Describe filter candles/candle filters/cartridge filters. (S. 02, 06; W. 01, 04)

☞ These are specially developed for very fine type of filtration.

Construction

– These are ceramic filters and are made of porcelain or kiesel guhr.
– These are cylindrical in shape with an opening which is connected to vacuum pump for carrying out the operation under reduced pressure.
– The candles are available in a range of different pore size.

Working

- The candle is placed in the solution to be filtered.

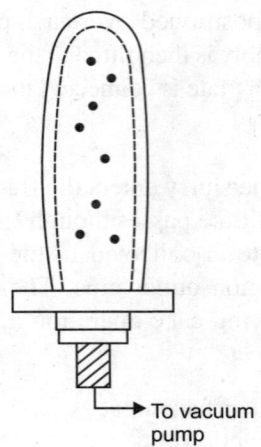

To vacuum
pump

- When vacuum is applied, the liquid will pass through the thick wall of the candle and get collected inside the candle from where it is removed.
- When it is used continuously, the candle gets blocked, thus it can be washed by passing water in reverse direction or by brushing the outer surface.

Advantages

1. It is used for microfiltration.
2. It is used for sterilisation of solutions.

Disadvantage

It absorbs the materials from aqueous solutions.

15 Describe metafilter. (S. 99, 04, 08; W. 97, 98, 01, 02, 04)

☞ Construction

(i) It consists of grooved, drainage rod on which a number of rings are packed, which are made up of stainless steel.

(ii) These rings have a number of semicircular projections on one surface and they are packed in such a way that the opening between the rings is about 0.2 mm.

Working

(i) The entire assembly is placed inside a pressure vessel, containing the liquid to be filtered.

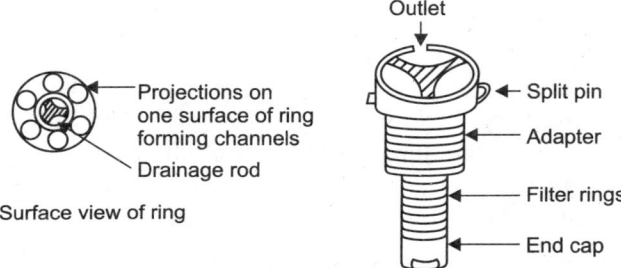

Surface view of ring

(ii) When vacuum is applied, liquid will flow from outside to inside.

(iii) In this way a metafilter can only be used as strainer for coarse particles.

(iv) The pack of rings acts as a base on which the true filter medium is supported.

Advantages

(i) It has considerable strength and hence, can withstand high pressure.

(ii) Corrosive liquids can be filtered.

(iii) Cake can be easily removed.

(iv) It is economical.

Application

It is useful for clarification of syrups, elixirs and parenteral solutions, oils, etc.

16 What is clarification? Explain various methods used for clarification. (S. 04)

☞ Clarification

It is the process of removal of relatively small amount of suspended solids (> 0.15%) present in the liquid without use of filter media.

This process is used in preparation of aromatic waters, fruit juices, syrups, honey or fixed oils.

Methods of Clarification

1. **Sedimentation and decantation:** The slurry or suspension is allowed to stand in a suitable container until the suspended matter settles down. The insoluble matter is the separated from clear liquid by decantation. Sedimentation can be increased by centrifugation.

2. **Colation/straining:** It is a crude filtration. Colation consists of separating large, visible particles of a solid from liquid by pouring mixture through a coarse cloth or porous substances like glass, wool, asbestos. The process of straining is to be repeated two or three times to get clear filtrate.

3. **Absorption and adsorption:** Soaking up or trapping of the foreign particles within the media is called absorption, while adherence of particles to the surface of media is called adsorption. Absorption and adsorption can be enhanced by adding filter aids.

4. **Siphoning:** It is a simple method of removal of clarified supernatant liquid. It works on the principle of siphoning.

5. **Temperature:** Increase in temperature of viscous liquid decreases viscosity, thus increases sedimentation and thus helps in clarification.

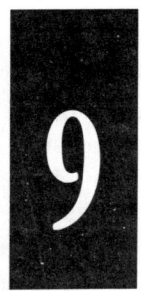

Extraction and Galenicals

1 Define the terms. (S. 02, 03; W. 01, 02, 07)

☞• **Extraction:** It is the process of removal of active constituents from crude drug by using a suitable solvent in which it is soluble.
• **Menstrum:** The solvent used for extraction is called menstrum, e.g. alcohol, water, chloroform, ether, light petroleum.
• **Marc:** The residue left after extraction is called marc.
• **Expression:** It means extraction carried out by mechanical means.
• **Galenicals:** The various preparations which are prepared by using extraction methods are called galenicals, e.g. infusions, decoction, tinctures, liquid extracts semisolid extracts.

2 Name various processes used for extraction. (S. 96, 97, 02; W. 99, 01, 02)

☞1. **Infusion:** It consists of pouring water over the drug and then allowed it to keep in contact with water for a period of usually 15 minutes, with occasionally stirring and finally filtering of liquids. The marc is not pressed. The boiling water is commonly used as a solvent, since it has a greater solvent action.
2. **Decoction:** It is the process in which drug is boiled with water for a stated period of usually 10 minutes. After boiling liquid is strained and water is passed through the content of the strainer to make the required volume.
3. **Maceration:** Maceration is the process of extraction in which the drug and whole quantity of menstrum is placed in closed

vessel and allowed to stand for 7 days with occasionally shaking. Thereafter liquid is strained, marc is pressed. The strained liquid and expressed liquid are combined and volume is not adjusted.

4. **Digestion:** It is the modified process of maceration in which drug and menstrum are heated throughout the extraction period to increase penetration power of the menstrum.

   The apparatus used for digestion is called digestor and temperature to be maintained is usually between 40 and 60°C.

5. **Percolation:** Percolation is the process in which a comminuted drug is extracted by the passage of suitable solvent through the column of a drug, packed in a percolator.

3 Write a note on solvents (menstrum) used for extraction. (S. 96, 07; W. 01, 07)

☞ Menstrum is a solvent used for the process of extraction.

• An ideal menstrum should possess following properties (S. 08; W. 05):

1. It should penetrate plant and animal tissues and cells.
2. It should dissolve active ingredient from crude a drug.
3. It should be nontoxic, noninflammable.
4. It should not cause degradation of dissolved substances.
5. It should be cheap and easily available.

Examples of Menstrum

A. Water

Water is a solvent for protein, colouring matter, gums, glycosides, sugars, alkaloidal salts, enzymes, etc.

Advantages

   (i) It is cheap.
   (ii) It has wide solvent action.
   (iii) It is nontoxic.
   (iv) It is noninflammable.

Disadvantages

   (i) It is not selective solvent.
   (ii) It is sensitive to bacterial and mould growth.
   (iii) It promotes hydrolysis of many substances.
   (iv) Large amount of heat is required to concentrate the product.

B. Alcohol (S. 04)

Alcohol is a solvent for alkaloids, glycosides, volatile oils and resins. Alcohol also dissolves many colouring matters, tannins, etc.

Advantages

(i) It is a selective solvent.

(ii) It is nontoxic.

(iii) It acts as a preservative.

(iv) It is neutral.

(v) It dissolves selective constituent of drug.

(vi) A small amount of heat is required to concentrate the product.

Disadvantages

(i) It is volatile.

(ii) It is inflammable.

(iii) It is costly.

4 Why is powdered drug used for extraction? OR Why comminution of drug prior to extraction is required?

☞ Because:

(i) In case of organised drug, the cell constituents are present in the fluid known as cell sap, in the form of solution or in colloidal state.

(ii) When the drug is dried, the constituents are precipitated or deposited in the cell structure. The dried cell sap becomes resistant to the action of menstrum.

(iii) The comminution of drug ruptures the cell sap and exposes the cell constituents to the action of menstrum.

(iv) Comminuted drug provides large surface area for penetration of the menstrum and effective extraction takes place.

5 Differentiate between the process for tinctures made from organised and unorganised drugs (maceration). (S. 96, 00, 03, 05; W. 99, 00, 07)

☞

Tinctures made from organised drug	Tinctures made from unorganised drug
1. The drug is placed with whole quantity of menstrum in a closed vessel	The drug is placed with only 4/5th volume of menstrum

Contd.

Tinctures made from organised drug	Tinctures made from unorganised drug
2. Maceration period is 7 days	Maceration period is 2 to 7 days
3. The marc is pressed	The marc is not pressed
4. The final volume is not adjusted	The final volume is adjusted
5. Examples:	Examples:
(i) Tincture of lemon	(i) Tincture of benzoin
(ii) Tincture of orange	(ii) Tincture of toluene

6 Distinguish between 'infusion' and 'decoction'.

☞

Infusion	Decoction
1. Cold or boiling water is used as menstrum	Drug is boiled in water
2. Drug having soft tissue is used	Drug of a hard tissue is used
3. Drug constituents may be volatile	Drug constituents should be nonvolatile
4. Final volume is not adjusted	Final volume is adjusted

7 What is percolation? Explain general stages involved in simple percolation process. (S. 97, 99, 00, 03, 07, 08, 09; W. 01, 02, 08)

☞ **Percolation**

Percolation is the process in which a comminuted drug is extracted by the passage of suitable solvent through the column of a drug packed in a percolator.

Simple Percolation

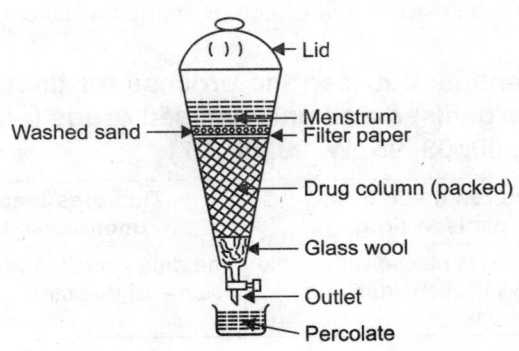

Stages Involved in Percolation

1. **Size reduction of drug:** The drug is powdered before packing into the percolator to provide uniform packing.

2. **Imbibition:** Imbibition means moistening of drug before packing into percolator. Imbibition is necessary because:

   (i) It allows the swelling of drug thus prevents blockage of percolator.

   (ii) It helps in uniform packing of drug.

   (iii) It helps to remove air from packed drug.

   (iv) It helps for passage of menstrum throughout the drug.

3. **Packing of drug in percolator:** Imbibed drug can be sieved to break any lump or masses. Moistened glass wool is placed at the bottom. Then whole quantity of drug is slowly packed into the percolator. A piece of filter paper is placed on the packed drug. Washed sand is then placed on the filter paper to prevent disturbance of top layer. Then sufficient quantity of menstrum is added into the percolator. When the liquid starts coming from the percolator, outlet is closed. Again sufficient menstrum is added.

4. **Maceration:** The drug is kept in contact with menstrum for 24 hours. The menstrum penetrates into the tissues of drug and dissolves active constituent.

5. **Collection of percolate:** After 24 hours outlet is opened and percolate is collected. Marc is pressed and added to percolate and volume is adjusted with menstrum.

6. **Clarification:** Finally to get clear solution, clarification is done.

8 Write a note on "soxhlation" or "Soxhlet's extraction" or "continuous hot percolation/extraction process". (S. 98, 03, 06, 08, 09; W. 96, 97, 99, 02, 03, 04, 06, 07)

☞ **Soxhlation**

When the active constituents of the crude drug are soluble in the menstrum or difficult to extract from the cells then the drug is treated with hot menstrum for considerable period of time. The apparatus is known as Soxhlet's extractor and process is known as soxhlation.

Soxhlet's Apparatus

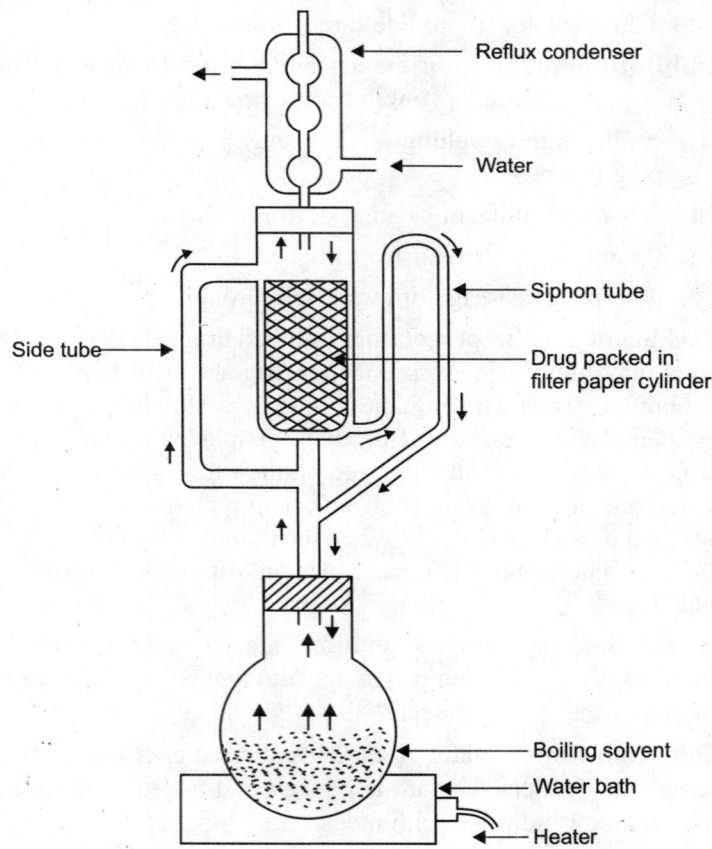

Apparatus

It consists of three main parts:

   (i) The flask containing boiling solvent.

   (ii) Soxhlet's extractor in which drug is packed.

      It has a side tube through which vapours of the solvent carried into the extractor. It has siphon tube which siphons over the extract from the Soxhlet's extractor to the flask.

   (iii) A condenser in which the vapours of the solvent are condensed and again converted into solvent.

Working

   (i) The drug to be extracted is packed in a paper cylinder made from filter paper and it is placed in the body of Soxhlet's extractor.

  (ii) The solvent is placed in the flask and then apparatus is fitted as shown in Figure.

 (iii) When solvent is boiled on heating the flask, it gets converted into vapours. These vapours enter into the condenser through the side tube and get condensed into hot liquid which falls on the column of the drug.

 (iv) When the extractor gets filled with solvent, the level of siphon tube also raises up to its top. The solvent containing active constituents of the drug in the siphon tube siphon over and run into the flask. The process of filling and emptying of extractor is continued until the drug is completely exhausted.

Advantages

1. Faster method.
2. Complete extraction of drug takes place.
3. Concentrated extract can be obtained.
4. Minimum requirement of menstrum.
5. Fireproof assembly.

Limitations/disadvantages

1. Method is not suitable for drugs which are sensitive to high temperature, e.g. enzymes, glycosides.
2. Only pure solvents can be used.
3. Gummy substances cannot be extracted by this method.

9 Define and classify ayurvedic dosage forms with examples. (S. 98, 99, 02, 03, 07; W. 98, 99, 00, 01, 02, 08)

☞ Ayurvedic Drugs

It means all medicines intended for internal or external use, or in the diagnosis, treatment, mitigation or prevention of disease or disorder in human beings or animals and are manufactured in accordance with the formulae described in authoritative books of Ayurveda specified in first schedule of the D&C Act, 1940.

Classification

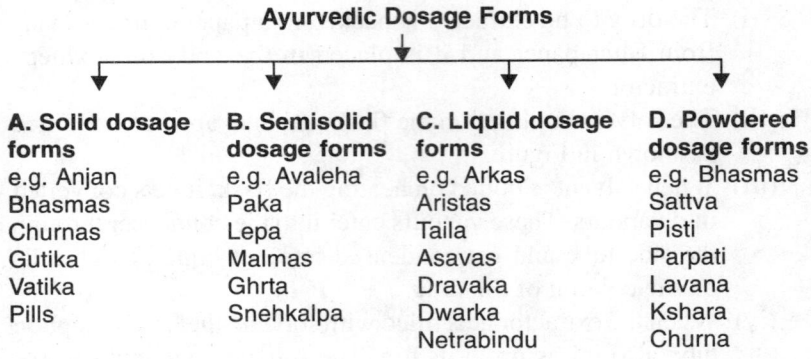

Ayurvedic Dosage Forms

A. Solid dosage forms	B. Semisolid dosage forms	C. Liquid dosage forms	D. Powdered dosage forms
e.g. Anjan	e.g. Avaleha	e.g. Arkas	e.g. Bhasmas
Bhasmas	Paka	Aristas	Sattva
Churnas	Lepa	Taila	Pisti
Gutika	Malmas	Asavas	Parpati
Vatika	Ghrta	Dravaka	Lavana
Pills	Snehkalpa	Dwarka	Kshara
		Netrabindu	Churna

10 **Define the terms:**

☞1. **Anjan (S. 98, 04, 05; W. 99, 08):** These are medicated finds powders intended to use in the eyes for their local effect.

2. **Netrabindu (S. 98, W. 99):** These are liquid preparations made by dissolving the specified form of drug in water or honey and used as eyedrops.

3. **Vatika/vati (S. 97):** Medicaments in the form of small tablet or pills are known as vati or vatika.

4. **Gutika (S. 97, 05):** These are large pills, prepared by converting the decoction of vegetable substances into thick consistency and then mixed with powdered medicine, raw sugar, honey.

5. **Avaleha (S. 97):** These are thick extracts of drug in which decoction of drug is prepared, strained and then boiled with sugar or honey to soft consistency.

6. **Asavas (S. 98, 04, 06; W. 03, 08):** These are medicated alcoholic liquids prepared by fermentation of raw vegetarian juice with honey or raw sugar for a period of 6 months.

7. **Aristas (S. 98, 06; W. 08):** These are weak alcoholic preparations prepared by making a decoction of drug and then it is fermented by using raw sugar or honey for a period of 7 to 10 days.

8. **Bhasmas (S. 97, 01, 04; W. 03, 08):** These are ashes prepared from vegetable and mineral substances and also from animal products.

9. **Churnas (S. 01, 04, 05):** These are powdered mixtures prepared by mixing dry mineral, animal or vegetable substances.

10. **Rasayanas/kupipakva:** These are preparations of metals containing mercury and are in the form of pills or tablets.

11. **Tailas:** Tailas are decoctions of vegetable drugs made with the addition of an oil.

12. **Sattva (S. 05):** Water extractable solid substance obtained from a drug is known as sattva.

13. **Lepa (S. 97):** These are semisolid preparations in the form of paste used for external application on the body.

14. **Dravakas:** These are the liquid preparations obtained from lavana or ksharas.

15. **Pakas (S. 97):** These are semisoid preparations of drugs prepared by addition of sugars, raw sugar and boiled with prescribed drug juice.

10

Evaporation

1 **What are various mechanisms of heat transfer? (S. 96, 02; W. 02)**

☞ **(i)** **Conduction:** In this mechanism heat transfer takes place by transmission of momentum of individual molecules, e.g. heat transfer in solids and liquids.

(ii) **Convection:** In this mechanism heat transfer takes place by actual motion of the particles, e.g. heat transfer in liquids.

(iii) **Radiation:** In this case heat transfer takes place through the space by means of electromagnetic waves which travel in a straight line at the speed of light, e.g. sun heat.

2 **Name various heat processes practised in pharmacy. (S. 96; W. 00)**

☞ **1.** **Sublimation:** It is the process in which solids get converted into vapours upon heating without formation of liquid and upon cooling the vapours get converted into solid.

2. **Desiccation:** Desiccation is the process of complete removal of adhered moisture from the substances.

3. **Exsiccation:** It is the process of removing water of crystallization of molecules under controlled conditions from the hydrated substance.

4. **Efflorescence:** It is the phenomenon in which substance looses water of crystallization molecules without heating.

5. **Deliquiscence:** It is the phenomenon in which the substances absorb water from surrounding and become damp and converted into liquid.
6. **Drying:** Drying means final removal of liquid from the solids with the help of heat.
7. **Evaporation:** It means free escape of vapours from the surface of the liquid below its boiling point.
8. **Distillation:** Distillation is the process of converting liquid into its vapours and reconverting it again into liquid by condensation.
9. **Calcination:** Calcination is the process in which inorganic substances are strongly heated to loose their volatile constituents with the formation of residue.
10. **Ignition:** It is the process in which substances completely burn out and ash is left behind. It is also called incineration.

3   **Define evaporation. Explain various factors affecting rate of evaporation. (S. 97, 98, 01, 03, 04, 05, 07; W. 97, 00, 01, 05, 06, 08)**

☞ **Evaporation**

Evaporation is a process of the free escape of vapour from the surface of liquid below its boiling point.

1. **Temperature:** When temperature increases the rate of evaporation increases.
2. **Temperature and time of evaporation:** Heating at high temperature for a short time is better than heating at low temperature for longer time.
3. **Temperature and moisture content:** Drugs containing moisture if heated at high temperature, undergo decomposition due to hydrolysis. To avoid this evaporation is done at low temperature and final drying is done at high temperature when a little moisture remains in the drug.
4. **Type of product required:** Upon evaporation of liquid concentrated liquid, semisolid and solid products are formed. Thus evaporation is done according to type of product required.
5. **Surface area of evaporator:** If surface area of evaporator is larger then rate of evaporation is faster.

6. **Vapour pressure of liquid:** If vapour pressure of the liquid is higher, then rate of evaporation is higher.
7. **Effect of concentration:** There is a possibility of formation of film on upper surface of liquid which decreases rate of evaporation. Thus constant stirring is required.

4 **Write a note on 'evaporating pan" (natural circulation evaporator). (S. 97, 98, 99, 03, 09; W. 98, 99)**

☞ **Evaporating Pan**

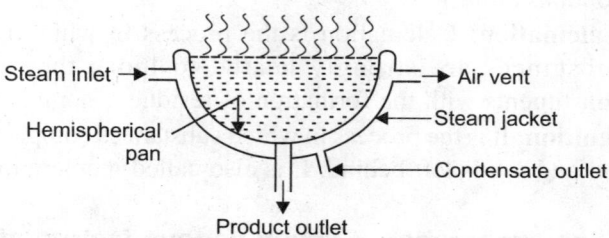

Construction and Working

  (i) It consists of a hemispherical pan made up of copper, stainless steel, etc.
 (ii) It is surrounded by steam jacket.
(iii) Hemispherical surface provides large surface area for evaporation.
(iv) The evaporating pan may be fixed or loose.
 (v) In case of fixed pans the product is taken out from the product outlet.

Advantages

  (i) It is very simple in construction.
 (ii) It is easy to clean and maintain.
(iii) It is economical.
(iv) It is very easy to handle.

Disadvantages

  (i) Possibility of decomposition of the product.
 (ii) Heating surface is limited.
(iii) Not suitable for heat-sensitive materials.
(iv) It is an open pan hence vapours produced may be dangerous to workers.

5 **Write a note on "evaporating still". (S. 00, 04, 05, 08; W. 98, 05)**

☞ This type of evaporator is commonly known as a "still" because evaporating pan is covered and connected to condenser.

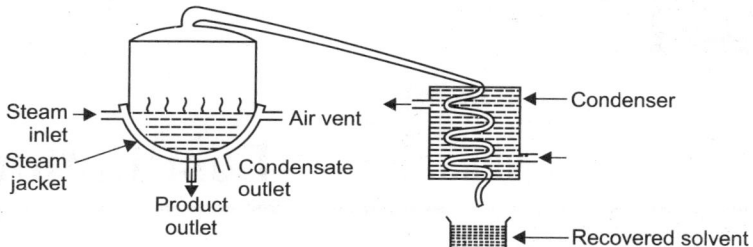

Construction and Working

1. In this case evaporating pan is covered and is connected to a condenser so that vapours are condensed into the liquid.
2. The pan is heated by means of steam jacket.
3. The vapours of the solvent are carried to the condenser where they get condensed. Thus costly solvent is recovered.
4. The concentrated product is taken out through the product outlet.

Advantages

(i) It is simple in construction.
(ii) Easy to maintain.
(iii) As vapours are condensed, the speed of evaporation increases.
(iv) Costly solvent can be recovered (alcohol).
(v) Operation can be conducted under reduced pressure.

Disadvantages

(i) Heating surface is limited.
(ii) Not suitable for thermolabile materials.
(iii) Coefficient heat transfer is poor.

Distillation

1. Define distillation. What are its types? (S. 96, 98; W. 01, 07)

☞ **Distillation**

Distillation is the process converting liquid into its vapours by heating and reconverting it again into liquid by condensing the vapours.

Types of Distillation

1. Simple distillation
2. Fractional distillation
3. Molecular distillation
4. Destructive distillation
5. Reflux distillation
6. Distillation under reduced pressure.

2. Differentiate between distillation and evaporation. (S. 02; W. 98, 99, 01, 02, 03)

☞

Distillation	Evaporation
1. It is the process of converting liquid into vapours and vapours again into liquid	It is the free escape of vapours from the surface of liquid
2. Liquid is heated at its boiling point	Liquid is heated below its boiling point
3. Vapours are formed throughout the liquid	Vapours are formed at the surface of a liquid
4. Vapours formed are condensed and collected	Vapours formed are not usually collected
5. It is used for isolation of volatile oils	It is used for preparation of concentrated liquid, soft extract and dry extract

3 **Define water for injection IP. Give method of preparation. (S. 00, 03; W. 97, 99, 02, 06)**

☞ **Definition**

It means the water which is free from volatile and nonvolatile impurities, microorganisms and pyrogens.

Method of Preparation

It is obtained by distillating potable water, purified water or distilled water from a neutral glass or metal still.

The first portion of distillate is rejected because it contains volatile impurities, i.e. dissolved O_2. The reminder is collected in the suitable containers previously rinsed with freshly distilled water and closed to avoid contamination. It contains no added substances.

12

Drying

1 Define drying. Give the pharmaceutical significance/ applications/importance of drying. (S. 98, 02, 04, 05, 09; W. 96)

☞ **Drying**

Drying means final removal of liquid from the solids with the help of heat.

Importance of Drying in Pharmacy

1. In pharma industry it is used in drying of granules, powders, etc.
2. Drying reduces weight of the substance, thus reduces the cost of transportation and storage.
3. Drying helps in preservation of drug.
4. Drying helps in the size reduction of drugs.
5. Drying improves flow property of drugs.
6. Drying is useful in manufacturing of different biological products.
7. Drying is useful in production of lactose, aluminium hydroxide, etc.

2 Name various equipment used in drying. (W. 99, 07, 08)

☞ (i) Tray dryer
(ii) Tunnel dryer
(iii) Spray dryer
(iv) Fludised bed dryer

(v) Rotary dryer   (vii) Freeze dryer

(vi) Vacuum dryer   (viii) IR dryer.

3 Explain tray dryer/compartment dryer. (S. 99, 06; W. 06, 07)

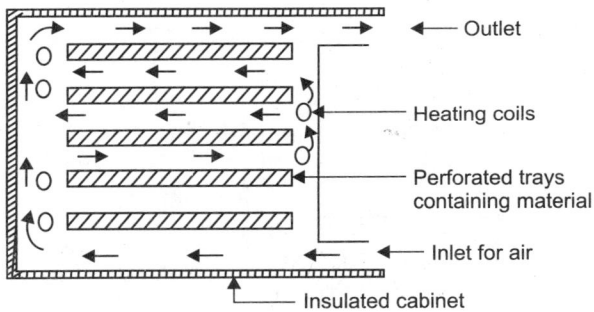

Construction

1. The simplest form of tray dryer is "laboratory oven".
2. It consists of insulated cabinet containing shelves.
3. It is heated by means of heaters fixed at the bottom.
4. It consists of trays on which the material to be dried is placed.
5. The trays have wire mesh bottom. The hot air passes over the surface of wet solids in the direction as shown in Figure.

Advantages

1. It can be used for drying of any type of material.
2. Temperature of drying can be controlled.
3. It is economical.
4. Easy to handle.

Disadvantages

1. Not suitable for heat-sensitive substances.
2. Large space is required for tray loading.
3. Labour cost is high.
4. Drying time is very long.
5. Drying is not uniform.

Applications/Uses

Tray dryers are used for drying of crude drugs, chemicals, powders and granules.

4 **Write a note on "fluidized bed dryer" (FBD). (S. 97, 98, 04, 07, 08, 09; W. 98, 00, 02, 03, 04, 08)**

☞

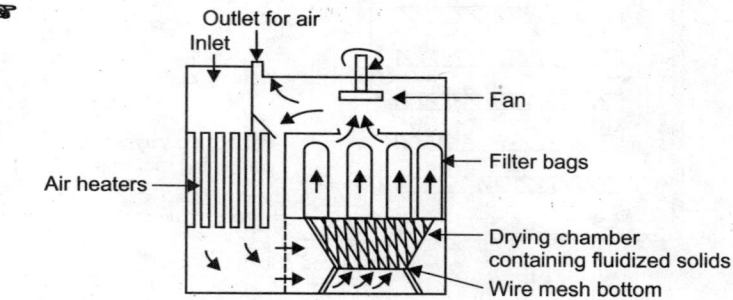

Construction and Working

1. The dryer consists of conical vessel with perforated bottom into which material is placed.
2. Filter bags are fitted to the conical vessel above which fan is fixed.
3. There is an inlet for air and outlet for air.
4. The fluidizing air stream is created by means of fan which is placed at the upper part of dryer.
5. Filtered and heated air then pass through powder bed.
6. The filter bags are provided to trap the fines produced during drying.

Advantages of Fluidized Bed Dryer (FBD)

1. High rate of drying.
2. Suitable for heat-sensitive materials.
3. Economical process.
4. Efficient and uniform drying.
5. It is mostly used for drying of granules.
6. Uniform temperature of drying can be maintained.
7. Product obtained is free flowing.

Disadvantages

1. High air velocity causes friction of particles.
2. High friction between particles generates electrostatic charges.
3. Due to turbulances fines are produced.

5 Write a note on vacuum dryer/vacuum oven.

☞

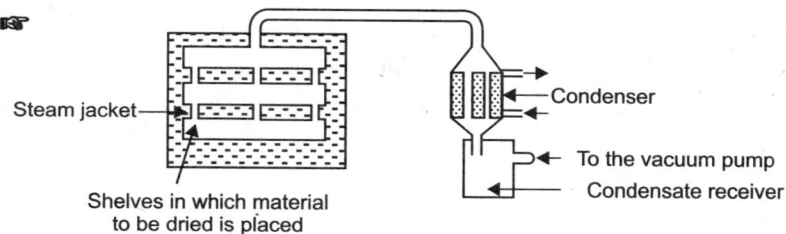

Steam jacket

Shelves in which material
to be dried is placed

Condenser

To the vacuum pump

Condensate receiver

Construction

It consists of steam-jacketed vessel made of strong material which can withstand the vacuum within the oven and pressure of the steam in the jacket. The door of oven provides tight sealing. The oven is connected to the vacuum pump through the condenser and receiver. Operating pressure is usually 0.03 to 0.06 bar at which the water boils at 25 to 35°C.

Advantages

1. Useful for heat-sensitive materials.
2. Valuable solvent can be recovered.
3. Helpful to obtain specific type of product.

Disadvantages

1. It has limited capacity.
2. It is costly method.

6 Write a note on spray dryer.

☞ **Construction**

1. It consists of cylindrical vessel having conical base.
2. There is a tangential inlet through which hot air enters and product is sprinkled through automiser.
3. Liquid feed inlet is located at the top and from bottom dry product is collected.

Working

(i) Spray dryer is used for drying the solutions and suspensions.

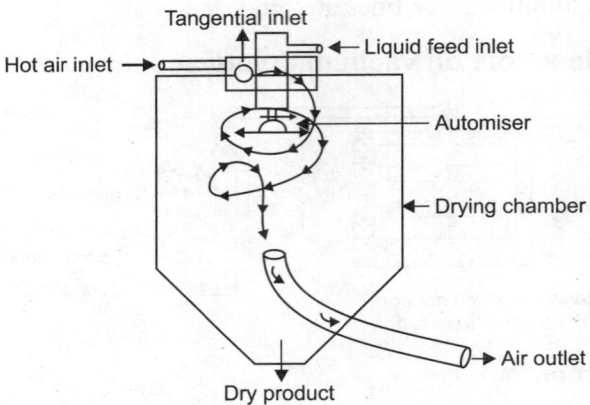

(ii) In the spray dryer the liquid to be dried is spread in the form of mist.

(iii) The minute droplets are readily evaporated and converted into solid particles which fall at the bottom of the chamber.

(iv) For drying the droplets hot air is introduced in the drying chamber through the tangential inlet and fine mist of liquid is produced with the help of automiser.

Advantages

(i) Useful for drying of heat-sensitive material.

(ii) The product obtained is fine and free flowing.

(iii) In encapsulation, i.e. coating of solids and liquid particles.

Disadvantages

(i) Skilled person is required to operate.

(ii) Method is costly.

7 What is freeze drying? Explain lyophilization/ lypophylization. (S. 97, 98, 00, 03, 05, 06, 09; W. 99, 04, 05, 06)

☞ It is also known as sublimation drying.

Lyophilization

It is the process of freeze drying in which the moisture present in the material is frozen and then removed by sublimation of ice, i.e. ice is converted into vapours.

Freeze Dryer

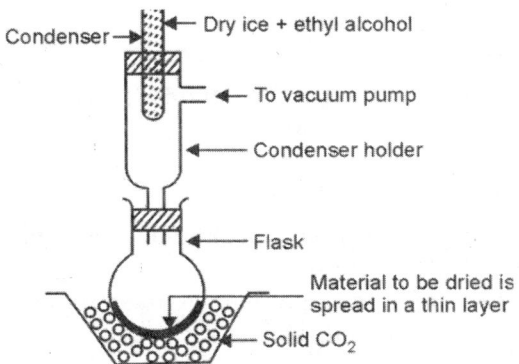

Construction and Working

Freeze dryer consists of four main parts:
1. A chamber for vacuum drying.
2. A vacuum source.
3. A heat source.
4. A vapour removal system.

Working

The material to be dried is frozen in a thin layer with the special type of freezing bottle. Spreading of material provides a large surface area for drying. The flask is connected to vacuum pump through the condenser. The temperature of condenser is maintained 20°C below the temperature of material to be dried. By creating vacuum in the flask the temperature and pressure conditions are set below the triple point value of water. Under such conditions if heat is supplied to the material it acts as a latent heat and sublimes the ice into vapour state. The vapours of water get condensed on the surface of condenser. The product obtained after freeze drying is light, porous and lyophilic in nature.

Advantages

1. Drying takes place at low temperature thus decomposition of product is minimized.
2. The product is more porous and light and readily soluble.
3. Oxidation of product can be minimized.
4. It is useful for drying of thermolabile materials.

Disadvantages

1. It is very slow process.
2. The process is very costly.
3. The product obtained is very hygroscopic therefore, requires special packaging conditions.

Pharmaceutical Applications

1. It is used for drying of biological products like plasma, serum, vaccines, enzymes, etc.
2. It is used for preservation of human tissue for research.
3. It is also used in food industry.

13

Sterilization

1 Define sterilization. Classify different methods of sterilization. (S. 97, 98, 99, 01, 04, 08; W. 96, 97, 99, 04, 05, 06, 08)

☞ **Sterilization**

Sterilization is the process of complete destruction of all microorganisms present in the system.

Methods of Sterilization

A. Physical methods
1. Dry heat sterilization, e.g. hot air oven.
2. Moist heat sterilization, e.g. autoclave.
3. Radiation sterilization:
    (a) By UV rays
    (b) Ionising radiations.

B. Chemical methods
1. Sterilization by heating with bactericide.
2. Gaseous sterilization.

C. Mechanical methods (sterilization by filtration)
1. Membrane filters.
2. Sintered glass filters.
3. Seitz filters.
4. Ceramic filters.

2 Define the terms. (S. 08)

☞(a) **Sterile product:** It means the product free from living organisms.

(b) **Sterility:** Sterility is a condition of freedom from living microorganisms.

(c) **Aseptic technique:** It is a controlled process or the technique which prevents contamination of microorganisms during the preparation and their testing.

(d) **Antiseptic:** A substance that prevents growth of microorganisms by inhibiting their activities without destroying them when applied for animate object.

(e) **Disinfectant:** A substance that destroys the microorganisms which when applied for inanimate object.

(f) **Disinfection:** A process that removes the infection potential by destroying microorganisms but not generally bacterial spores.

(g) **Bactericide:** The substance that kills bacteria is called bactericide.

(h) **Bacteriostatic:** The substance that stops the growth of bacteria.

(i) **Viricide:** A substance that kills viruses.

(j) **Germicide:** A substance that kills germs.

3 Differentiate between sterilization and disinfection. (S. 04, 05, 09)

☞

Sterilization	Disinfection
1. It is the process of complete destruction of all microorganisms present in the system	It is the process that removes the infection potential by microorganisms
2. It case of sterilization spores are also destroyed	Spores are not destroyed
3. Sterilization is done by using any of the physical/chemical/mechanical methods	Disinfection is done by using any of the disinfectants

4 What is aseptic technique? Give the design/precautions to be taken during aseptic processing (sterile area). (S. 99, 02, 06; W. 99, 03, 04, 05)

☞ **Aseptic Technique**

It is the technique which prevents contamination of microorganisms during the preparation of products and their testing.

Design/Construction/Requirements/Precautions of Aseptic Area

1. Aseptic area should be away from crowdy area.
2. Windows must be provided with glass.
3. Laminar air flow should be provided.
4. Doors should have air-lock system to prevent sudden rush of air inside.
5. Aseptic area should have positive pressure.
6. Ceiling walls and floors should be smooth and easily washable.
7. There should be minimum counters and should be made up of stainless steel.
8. The air in the aseptic area should be filtered through HEPA.
9. Walls should have glazed tiles.
10. UV lamps should be provided.
11. All the equipment and apparatu should be sterilized.
12. The movements in the aseptic area must be minimum.
13. Sufficient space should be provided to the workers in aseptic area.
14. The person entering the room should enter through air-lock system and should wear sterile gown, cap, masks, gloves and footwares.
15. The person working in aspetic area should be free from any disease or disorder.
16. Regular medical checkup of workers is necessary.

5 Write a note on "hot air oven"/ dry heat sterilization. (S. 05; W. 97, 98, 99, 06, 08)

☞ Hot air oven works on the principle of killing the organism by dry heat at 150 to 170°C for one hour.

Dry heat kills microorganisms by oxidation of cell proteins.

Construction and Working

1. It is a double-walled chamber made up of stainless steel or aluminium.
2. Insulation of asbestos is filled between two walls to prevent heat loss.
3. Door is also double-walled with gasket on its inner side.
4. Two or three perforated shelves are fixed inside it.

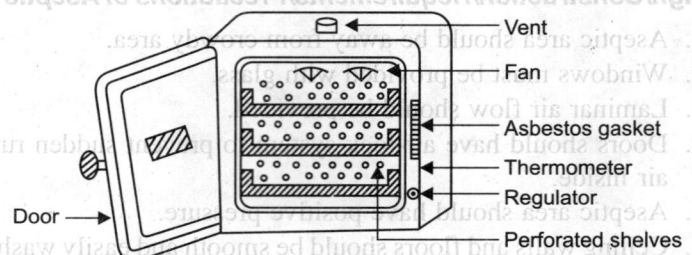

5. Electric fan is fitted inside to have uniform circulation of heat.
6. Heating coil is fitted at the bottom.
7. Temperature is regulated with thermometer and thermostatic device.
8. The material to be sterilized is placed on the shelves.
9. The temperature and time are set.
10. After complete sterilization, switch off the current.
11. Cool the oven for half an hour. Then open and take the materials.

Precautions to be Taken

1. Glass material must be wrapped with filter paper.
2. Containers must be plugged with nonabsorbent cotton wool.
3. Do not overload the materials.
4. Keep sufficient space between the articles.
5. Do not place the materials on the floor of the oven.

Advantages

1. Suitable for equipment like glass, steel utensiles.
2. Useful for oily materials and powders.
3. Operations are easy.
4. Suitable methods for sterilization of assembled equipment like glass syringes, metal equipment, etc.

Disadvantages

1. Not suitable for surgical dressings.
2. Not suitable for rubber, plastic goods.
3. Electricity is required.

Applications/Uses

1. Mainly used for sterilization of glasswares, such as flask, pipettes, tubes, bottles, mortars and pastles, etc.

2. It is used for sterilization of powders such as kaolin, talc, etc.
3. It is used for sterilization of injection containing fixed oil as a vehicle, e.g. injection of testosterone.
4. It is used for sterilization of metal equipment like scalpels, spatulas, blades, scissors, glass syringes.

6 Write a note on "moist heat sterilization"/"autoclave". (S. 96, 98, 01, 04, 07, 09; W, 01, 03, 04, 06, 07, 08)

☞• Steam has more penetration power than dry heat.
• Moist steam penetrates the spores and capsules of bacteria, ruptures it and thus kills bacterial spores.
• "Autoclave" is an instrument used for "moist heat sterilization".

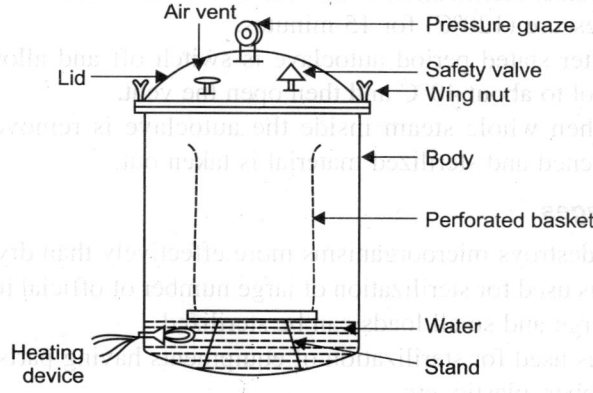

Autoclave

Principle

In the autoclave saturated steam under pressure is used which causes destruction of microorganisms and spores.

Construction

1. It consists of strong metallic chamber made up of stainless steel.
2. It has cover, consists of air vent, pressure gauze and safety valve.
3. Rubber gasket is fitted inside to make autoclave airtight.
4. Wing nut and bolts help to close the lid.
5. A perforated basket is kept on the stand.
6. Heat device is fitted at the bottom.

Working

1. Add sufficient water in the autoclave.
2. The perforated basket with materials to be sterilized is kept on the stand.
3. Close the lid and tight the wing nuts.
4. Autoclave is switched on to heat the water.
5. The air vent is opened and safety valve is set at the required pressure.
6. When the steam starts coming out from the vent, it is allowed to come for 5 minutes and then closed.
7. Steam pressure starts increasing. When desired pressure is attained it is kept constant for the stated period.
8. Usually sterilization in autoclave is carried out at 15 IBS/inch^2 pressure (120°C) for 15 minutes.
9. After stated period autoclave is switch off and allowed it to cool to about 40°C and then open the vent.
10. When whole steam inside the autoclave is removed, lid is opened and sterilized material is taken out.

Advantages

1. It destroys microorganisms more effectively than dry heat.
2. It is used for sterilization of large number of official injections.
3. Large and small loads can be sterilized.
4. It is used for sterilization of equipments having parts made of rubber, plastic, etc.
5. Method is applicable for wide variety of materials.

Disadvantages/Limitations

1. Not suitable for sterilization of powders and oils.
2. Not suitable for materials which cannot withstand temperature more than 115°C for 30 minutes and above.

Applications

1. It is used for sterilization of surgical dressings, surgical instruments.
2. The container and closures can be sterilized by autoclave.
3. It is used for the sterilization of a majority of official injections.
4. It is used for sterilization of articles made of rubber, plastic, glass.

7 Write a note on "radiation sterilization"/"cold sterilization". (S. 96, 97, 00, 02, 03; W. 96, 04)

☞ Radiation sterilization is of two types:

A. Sterilization by UV Rays (S. 08)

– Antimicrobial activity of ultraviolet rays depends upon its wavelength and it is maximum at 265 nm.
– Sunlight contains UV rays of long wavelength.
– UV rays for sterilization are produced by passing a low current at high voltage through mercury vapours in evacuated glass tube.

Advantages/Applications

1. It is used for sterilization of air in hospital.
2. It is used for sterilization of the area in which aseptic technique is carried out.
3. It is used for sterilization of thermolabile substances before packing.

Disadvantages

1. UV rays have low penetration power, so it is not applicable for sterilization of packed pharmaceuticals.
2. UV rays are less effective if humidity is high.
3. Accumulation of dust/grease on the UV lamp reduces its radiations.
4. Regular cleaning of lamp is required.
5. UV light is harmful to the workers.

B. Sterilization by Ionising Radiations

– Ionising radiations are X-rays and gamma rays.
– These rays are toxic to bacterial cells and destroy the cell nucleus.
– γ-rays are produced from radioisotopes like cobalt-60.
– Ionizing radiations are more efficient than UV rays.
– The material to be sterilized is packed in the final container and exposed to the ionizing radiations for specified period.

Advantages

1. γ-rays have high penetration power thus materials in final container can be sterilized.

2. The method is suitable for all types of materials like dry, moist and frozen.

3. Some bacterial vaccines and viral vaccines are sterilized by this method.

4. Large quantity of material can be sterilized.

5. Rise in temperature is negligible.

Disadvantages

1. Once the process is started, it cannot be stopped.

2. Radiations are harmful to workers.

3. It may cause undesirable changes in medicament like colour, solubility.

4. The plant is very costly.

Applications

1. This method is mainly used for sterilization of plastic syringes, hypodermic needles, surgical blades and adhesive dressings.

2. It can be used for sterilization of the thermolabile drugs.

3. It is used for sterilization of bone and tissue transplants, plastic tubing catheter and sutures.

8 Write a note on "chemical method of sterilization". (S. 09)

☞ It is of two types:

A. Sterilization by Heating with Bactericide (S. 99, 01)

This method is based on the fact that bactericides are more effective at high temperature than low temperature. In this method preparation containing stated amount of bactericide is heated in the final container in boiling water at 90–100°C for 30 minutes.

IP permits the following bactericides:

1. For injections:
   (i) Chlorocresol 0.1% w/v
   (ii) Phenylmercuric nitrate/acetate 0.002% w/v.

2. For eyedrops:
   (i) Benzalkonium chloride 0.01%
   (ii) Phenylmercuric nitrate/acetate 0.002% w/v.

B. Gaseous Sterilization (S. 96, 03, 04, 07; W. 96, 01, 02, 04, 05)

Gaseous sterilization means destruction of all living microorganisms with a chemical in gas or vapour state, e.g. formaldehyde, ethylene oxide, β-propiolactone.

(a) **Formaldehyde:** It is an alkylating agent. It has been used for fumigation of rooms and hospital blankets.

(b) **Ethylene oxide:** It is a colourless gas. It is highly inflammable. The sterilization with the mixture of ethylene oxide and inert gas is done in a chamber which is heated to the desired degree of temperature. The material tube sterilized is packed in the chamber and treated with sterilizing mixture for the stated period.

Advantages

1. It is suitable for heat-sensitive substances.
2. Because of good penetration power it can be used for sterilization of prepacked drugs.

Disadvantages

1. It is a slow method.
2. Running cost is high.
3. A lot of precautions are required while handling it.

Applications

1. It is used for sterilization of thermolabile materials like rubber and plastic items.
2. Used for the sterilization of syringes, needles, metallic equipments, etc.

C. β-Propiolactone

It is a latest sterilizing agent and used for sterilization of operation theatres and aseptic rooms.

9 Explain "sterilization by filtration" (mechanical method). (S. 99, 08; W. 00, 08)

☞• It is a nonthermal method widely used in pharma industry for heat-sensitive medicaments.

• For this purpose solution of substance is passed through bacteria-proof filter and sterile filtrate is collected in sterile receiver.

- Commonly used bacteria-proof filters are:
  1. Membrane filter.
  2. Ceramic filter.
  3. Seitz filter.
  4. Sintered metal filter.
  5. Sintered glass filter.

Precautions Required for Sterilization by Filtration

1. Whole apparatus must be sterile.
2. An aseptic technique should be followed to prevent contamination.
3. There should be minimum exposure of filtrate to atmosphere.
4. The filter should be very fine to trap all bacteria.

Stages Involved in Filtration Sterilization

1. Filtration of solution through the previously sterilized bacteria-proof filter.
2. Aseptic transfer of filtrate into the final sterile container.
3. Aseptic sealing of final container.
4. Testing of sample for sterility.

Applications/Advantages

1. Suitable for sterilization of heat-sensitive medicaments and substances like blood products, insulin, enzymes.
2. All types of bacteria whether living or dead bodies are removed.
3. Both clarification and sterilization are done side by side.

Disadvantages

1. The method is not reliable. Therefore, sterility test is always necessary.
2. Aseptic technique is necessary.
3. Suspension and oily preparations cannot be sterilized.
4. Careful handling and skilled worker are necessary.

10 Describe the "test for sterility". (S. 98, 05; W. 98)

☞ Principle

Test for sterility is conducted to ensure that the sterilization process is effectively carried out.

Sterility test is based on the principle that if bacteria/fungi are placed in the nutritive media at desired temperature and pH, the organisms will grow and its presence can be indicated by turbidity in the original clear medium.

Methods for Sterility Testing

A. Membrane Filtration Method

In this method sample is filtered through sterile membrane filter. After filtration, the membrane is removed aseptically. This membrane is transferred into 100 ml of culture media and incubated at 20 to 25°C for about 7 days.

Observation

If turbidity appears on the culture media/membrane then sample is not sterile.

B. Direct Inoculation Method

In this method specified quantity of sample is transferred into the sterile culture media and mixed well. It is incubated for not less than 7 days.

Observation

After incubation, culture medium is observed.
1. If there is turbidity in the culture medium, it indicates the growth of microorganisms and the sample does not pass test for sterility.
2. If the culture medium is clear it indicates absence of micro-organisms and sample passes the test for sterility.

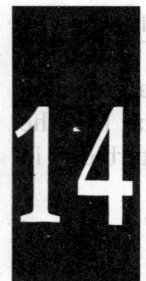

Processing of Tablet

1 Define tablet. Give advantages and disadvantages of tablet. (S. 98, 99, 02, 07, 08, 09; W. 96, 01)

☞ **Tablet**

Tablets are solid, flat or biconvex disc-shaped, prepared by compressing a drug or mixture of drug with or without diluents.

Advantages/Merits

1. Tablets are easy for administration.
2. Tablets are easy to dispense.
3. Tablets are stable dosage forms.
4. Tablets give accuracy of dosage.
5. Masking of taste is possible by tablet coating.
6. Rapid disintegration, dissolution and onset of action.
7. They are light in weight.
8. Packaging and transportation of tablets is cheapest.
9. Tablets are economical dosage forms.
10. They can be formulated as a sustained dosage form.

Disadvantages/Demerits

1. Tablets are difficult to be swallowed by children and ill patients.
2. Some drugs are difficult to compress into tablet due to their low density.
3. Bitter and nauseous drugs require coating or encapsulation.
4. The drugs with poor wetting and slow dissolution property are difficult to convert into tablets.

2 Classify tablets. (S. 96, 97, 99, 01, 06, 09; W. 01, 06, 08)

☞ **Classification/Types of Tablets**

A. Tablets Ingested Orally

1. Compressed tablets.
2. Multiple compressed tablets.
3. Multilayered tablets.
4. Sustained action tablets.
5. Enteric-coated tablets.
6. Sugar-coated tablets.
7. Film-coated tablets.
8. Chewable tablets.

B. Tablets Used in Oral Cavity

1. Buccal tablets.
2. Sublingual tablets.
3. Lozenge tablets.
4. Dental cones.

C. Tablets Used by other Routes

1. Implants.
2. Vaginal tablets.

D. Tablets Used to Prepare Solution

1. Solution tablets.
2. Effervescent tablets.
3. Dispensing tablets.
4. Hypodermic tablets.
5. Tablet triturates.

3 Write a note on additives/excipients/adjuvants used in tablets. (S. 97, 98, 99, 02, 08; W. 97, 99, 00, 02, 04, 07, 08)

☞ 1. **Diluents:** When quantity of medicament in each tablet is very small then to make a tablet diluent is necessary, e.g. lactose, sucrose, dextrose, starch.

2. **Granulating agents:** These are used to convert fine powder into granules. Granulating agent provides proper moisture to convert fines into granules, e.g. water, alcohol, starch paste.

3. **Binding agents/binders:** These are used in granulation to provide proper strength to the granules, e.g. gum acacia, gum tragacanth, gelatin, starch paste, sucrose.

4. **Disintegrating agents:** These agents cause breakdown of tablet into small pieces. When medicament is insoluble in water, a disintegrating agent is required, e.g. starch, cellulose, alginates.

5. **Lubricants/glidants:** These are added to improve flow property of granules and to prevent sticking of materials to die and punches, e.g. talc, magnesium stearate, boric acid, calcium stearate.

6. **Adsorbents/adsorbing agents:** These are used to adsorb volatile oils, liquid extracts and tinctures, e.g. magnesium carbonate, kaolin, starch.

7. **Colouring agents:** These provide attractive colour to the tablet, e.g. amaranth, indigocarmine.

8. **Flavouring agents:** These provide pleasant flavour to the tablet, e.g. mentha oil, peppermint oil.

9. **Sweetening agents:** These mask the bitter taste of the tablet, e.g. sucrose, lactose.

4 **What are various steps involved during manufacturing of compressed tablets? (S. 06; W. 04, 07)**

☞ 1. Preparation of granules for compression:
   (a) Weighing the ingredients.
   (b) Mixing the powdered ingredients and excipients.
   (c) Converting the mixed ingredients into granules.
2. Compression of granules into tablets.
3. Coating of tablets.
4. Evaluation of tablets.

5 **What are different methods of preparation of granules?**

☞ **Granulation Methods**

(a) Moist/wet granulation.
(b) Dry granulation.
(c) Slugging/preliminary compression method.

(a) Moist/Wet Granulation (S. 96, 04, 05)

1. All powdered medicaments are mixed together.
2. By adding granulating agent powdered ingredients are converted into coherent mass.
3. This coherent mass is then passed through sieve no. 8 or 10.
4. The wet granules are dried in the oven below 60°C.
5. The dried granules are again passed through sieve no. 20 to obtain uniform-sized granules.
6. Then lubricants and remaining part of the disintegrating agents are added to the granules and thus granules are ready for compression.

(b) Dry Granulation (S. 96, 98, 99, 00, 01; W. 98, 06)

This method is used when certain medicaments are available in crystalline form or in the form of granules. Such medicaments are passed through sieve no. 20 or any other specified sieve and then mixed with any additional excipient. The resulting mixture is ready for compression, e.g. aspirin, sodium bromide, potassium chlorate.

(c) Slugging/Granules Prepared by Preliminary Compression (S. 96, 98, 00, 01; W. 98)

This method is used if drug is unstable in presence of moisture.

1. In this process the dry powder is compressed into large tablets or "slugs".
2. These slugs are broken into small pieces which are passed through specified sieve to collect the granules of suitable size.
3. A lubricating agent and a disintegrating agent are mixed with these granules and granules are ready for compression.

6 Why are granules preferred for compression than powders? (S. 00, 03, 07; W. 02, 04)

☞ Granules are preferred for compression than powders because:

1. Granules have uniform distribution of active ingredients.
2. Granules have spherical shape.
3. Granules give sufficient strength to tablets.
4. Granules of different sizes produce good die filling.
5. Granules are packed down easily and produce hard tablet.
6. Granules are heavier thus do not blow out of die cavity.

7 Explain various defects/problems in manufacturing (processing) of tablets. (S. 96, 97, 98, 05; W. 97, 99, 03, 05, 06, 07)

☞ **(a) Capping**

It means partial or complete removal of top or bottom portion of the tablet.

Causes/Reasons

1. Excessive fines in the granules which entrap air in the tablet.
2. Defective punches and dies.
3. High speed of the tablet machine.
4. The granules are too dry.
5. The punches are not set properly.
6. High degree of compression.

Remedy

1. Reduce the percentage of fines in granules.
2. Defective punches should be replaced.
3. Regulate the speed of the tablet machine.
4. Maintain desired moisture in the granules.
5. Set the punches and dies properly.
6. Regulate the pressure and reduce degree of compression.

(b) Picking and Sticking

"Picking" means the upper punch removes/picks up the material from the upper surface of the tablet.

"Sticking" means the material sticks to the walls of die cavity and punches.

Causes/Reasons

1. Use of scratched dies and punches.
2. Presence of moisture in the granules.
3. Use of small quantity of lubricant.
4. Excess of powder in the granules.
5. Defects in formulation.

Remedy

1. Use new set of die and punches.
2. Reduce moisture in the granules (dry the granules).

3. Increase quantity of lubricant.
4. Reduce percentage of powder in the granules.
5. Formulation should be checked.

(c) Mottling

"Mottling" means unequal distribution of colour on the surface of a coloured tablet.

Reasons/Causes

1. Migration of dye in the granules during the process of drying.
2. Use of different coloured medicaments and additives.
3. Non-uniform drying of granules.

Remedy

1. Drying of granules at a low temperature.
2. Using the dye which masks the colour of all ingredients.

(d) Weight Variation

It means the tablets do not have uniform weight.

Causes/Reasons

1. Granules are not uniform in size.
2. Excess of powder in the granules.
3. No proper mixing of lubricant.
4. No uniform flow of granules from hopper to die.
5. Due to change in capacity of die during compression.
6. Variation in speed and vibration of machine.

Remedy

1. Make granules of uniform size.
2. Reduce % of powder in the granules.
3. Uniform mixing of lubricant.
4. Maintain uniform flow of granules.
5. Reduce vibrations of machine and control variation in speed.

(e) Hardness Variation

- It means tablets do not have uniform hardness.
- The causes of hardness variation are similar to weight variation.
- By adjusting distance between punches and volume of material entering the die, hardness variation can be controlled.

(f) Double Impression

- This defect occurs when the lower punch has a monogram.
- This defect occurs because of improper movement of lower punch.
- This defect can be removed by controlling undesirable movement of the lower punch.

(g) Lamination

It refers to breakdown of tablet into two or more layers.

(h) Chipping

Chipping refers to coming off of a small portion of tablet.

8 Explain why tablets are coated? Name types of coating. (S. 97, 99, 03, 06; W. 97, 98, 00, 01, 08)

☞ The tablets are coated for the following reasons:
1. To mask the unpleasant taste of tablet.
2. To control the site of dissolution.
3. To protect the drug from atmospheric effects like air, moisture, etc.
4. To make the tablet attractive.
5. To provide susbtained release action of drug.
6. To produce pharmaceutically superior products.
7. To prevent interaction of incompatible ingredients.
8. To convert liquid into free-flowing solids.

Types of Tablet Coating

1. Film coating, e.g. polyethylene glycol, hydroxy propyl methyl cellulose.
2. Sugar coating, e.g. plane/coloured syrup.
3. Enteric coating, e.g. shellac, cellulose acetate phthalate.
4. Compression coating
5. Controlled release coating.

9 Write a note on "sugar coating of tablets". (S. 06; W. 03, 06, 07, 08)

☞ Sugar coating is an art and requires skilled workers.
It is done by pan coating method.

Stages Involved during Sugar Coating

1. **Sieving:** The fine powder and broken pieces of tablet are removed by sieving.

2. **Sealing:** It involves layering of tablet by waterproof materials like shellac, cellulose acetate phthalate. The material is dissolved in water/solvent and spread over the rotating tablets on the pan, which causes evaporation of volatile solvent and thin coat of waterproof material remain, i.e. sealing.

3. **Subcoating:** In this stage several coats of sugar and other materials such as gelatin, acacia, etc. are given to round off tablet and helps to build up the tablet size. During subcoating dusting powder is sprinkled to prevent sticking of tablets.

4. **Syrup coating:** This is done to give sugar coat and colour to the tablet. Colouring materials and opacifying agents are also added to the syrup.

5. **Finishing:** At the end of the process 3–4 coats of syrup are applied in rapid succession. Cold air is circulated to dry each coat. Finishing provides smooth and hard surface to tablet.

6. **Polishing:** Polishing pan is made of canvas cloth. Tablets are placed in rotating polishing pan. Before polishing, layer of bees wax is applied.

10 Explain "film coating of tablets". (S. 96, 06; W. 00, 04)

☞ Film coating means coating by means of film forming agents such as hydroxy ethyl methyl cellulose, polyethylene glyco-400, carbowax, PVC, CMC, ethyl cellulose, etc.

Method of Film Coating of Tablets

1. The tablets are placed in the coating pan.
2. The speed of the pan is so adjusted that the tablets tumble in pan.
3. Hot air is blown in.
4. The film coating solution is added.
5. After each addition, dusting powder is sprinkled, if necessary.
6. In the end, the coated tablets are dried off.

Advantages of Film Coating

1. It is less time-consuming technique.
2. Not much labour is required.

3. No significant increase in tablet weight or size.
4. No effect on disintegration of tablet.
5. The product cost is low because of cheaper coating material.
6. Film coating protects the drug from air, moisture, light, etc.
7. Coating is resistant to cracking and chipping.
8. No waterproofing is required before actual film coating.
9. The tablets become elegant.

11 What is enteric coating? Why is it necessary? Explain its method. (S. 99, 00, 01, 06, 07; W. 96, 99, 01, 03, 04)

☞ "Enteric coating" means coat is applied to the tablet so that tablet shall disintegrate in the intestine and not in the stomach.

The Tablets are Enteric Coated Because

1. Some medicaments produce severe irritation in the stomach.
2. The action of medicament is required in the intestine.
3. Some medicaments get destroyed by acidic medium of the stomach.
4. Drug absorption is better in the intestine.
5. Delayed action is needed.
6. When sustained action of drug is required.

Materials Used for Enteric Coating

1. Shellac.
2. Cellulose acetate phthalate.
3. Synthetic resins.
4. Salol.

Properties of an Ideal Enteric Coating Material

1. Resistant to gastric fluid.
2. Nontoxic in the required quantity.
3. Economical.
4. Ease of application.
5. Compatible with drug on which coating is done.
6. Formation of continuous film.
7. Film should not change on aging.
8. Should readily dissolve in intestinal fluids.

Method of Entering Coating

1. On large scale enteric coating is done in rotating pan.
2. The tablets to be coated are taken into the pan.
3. The pan is rotated with a sufficient speed.
4. First waterproofing of the tablet is done by solutions of shellac.
5. Then enteric coating solution is sprayed over the tablets rotated in the coating pan.
6. The hot air is blown into the pan to evaporate the organic solvent.
7. The process is repeated a number of times till the required number of coatings are done.

12 Give the difference between 'pan coating and press coating'.

Pan coating	Press coating
1. The solution of coating material is used	Coat is used
2. Tablets must be hard to withstand tumbling with the coating pan	Tablets need not to be hard
3. It is a batch process	It is continuous process
4. It is skilled process	It is mechanical process
5. Embossing of tablet is not possible	Embossing of tablet is possible

13 Name and explain common defects in film coating. (S. 96)

1. **Blistering:** A film surface shows number of uneven spots called blisters.
2. **Wrinkling:** It means formation of wrinkles on surface of film by improper drying.
3. **Orange peel:** It means formation of film surface like orange peel due to rapid drying.
4. **Sweeting:** It means presence of an oily film or liquid droplet on the surface of the coat.
5. **Flaking:** It means removal of coating material like a flakes.
6. **Blooming:** If the product is processed under high humidity conditions, there is a formation of dull film known as blooming.

7. **Spotting:** It means formation of spotted area on the surface of tablet film because of migration of dyes, plasticizers, etc.

8. **Bridging:** It means there is a lack of adhesion of the film to the tablet surface showing bridge-like appearance.

14 Write a note on microencapsulation. (S. 01, 06; W. 00, 04, 05)

☞ **Microencapsulation**

It is the technique in which a thin coating is applied on the particles of solids, liquids, resulting in formation of microcapsules ranging from 5 µm to 5 mm.

Microencapsulation is used to:

1. Mask the taste of bitter drugs.
2. Formation of sustained release dosage form.
3. Separation of incompatible materials.
4. Protection of drugs against moisture, oxygen, etc.
5. Conversion of liquid to solids, etc.

The materials used for microencapsulation are gelatin, PVC, ethyl cellulose, shell, etc.

Microencapsulation is generally carried out by coacervation or phase inversion technique.

15 Name various official and unofficial tests for evaluation of tablet quality control tests/pharmacopoeial tests (standardisation tests). (S. 98, 00, 01, 02, 06, 08, 09; W. 96, 99, 01, 05, 06)

☞ **Evaluation of Tablets**

A. Official Tests

1. Shape of tablets
2. Appearance
3. Content of active ingredient in tablets
4. Uniformity of weight (weight variation)
5. Uniformity of contents
6. Disintegration test
7. Dissolution test

B. Unofficial Tests

1. Hardness test
2. Friability test

16 Write a note on 'weight variation' of tablets. (S. 01, 04; W. 01)

☞ Every individual tablet in a batch should be uniform in weight but a small variation in the weight of individual tablets occurs. Therefore, little variation is allowed in the weight of a tablet by pharmacopoeia.

Average weight of tablet	% Deviation
1. 80 mg or less	10
2. More than 80 mg and less than 250 mg	7.5
3. 250 mg or more	5

Weigh 20 tablets selected at random and determine their average weight. Not more than 2 tablets may deviate from the average weight.

17 Write a note on "disintegration test" for tablets. (S. 96, 98, 00, 04; W. 96, 97, 99, 01, 05, 08)

☞ • Disintegration: Disintegration of a tablet means to break the tablet into smaller particles after swallowing.
  • Disintegration time: Time required to disintegrate the tablet is called disintegration time.
  • This test is performed to determine whether the coated or uncoated tablets disintegrate within the prescribed time, when placed in the liquid medium under prescribed experimental conditions.
  • Rate of disintegration depends upon the nature of drug and hardness of the tablet.
  • In general, pharmacopoeia prescribed a limit of 15 minutes for most of the tablets.

The Official Disintegration Test as per IP 1985

• **Disintegration Test Apparatus**

It consists of:
  1. A rigid basket-rack assembly supporting 6 cylindrical glass tubes 77.5 mm long, 21 mm in diameter and 2 mm in thickness.
  2. Lower size of the tube is covered with a stainless steel mesh of 2 mm apertures.

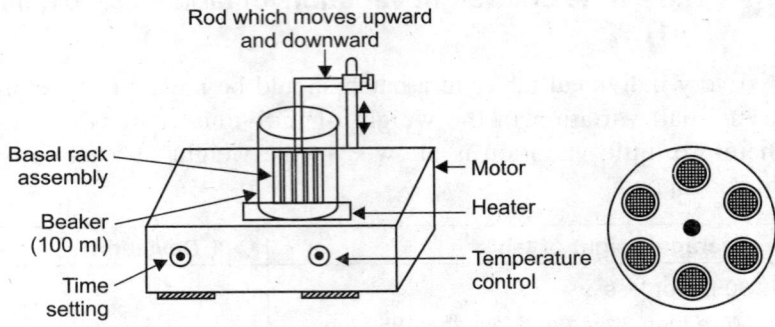

Disintegration test apparatus

3. Metal rod is fixed to the centre of the basket and attached to a mechanical device which moves up and down through a distance of 50 to 60 mm at frequency of **28 to 32 cycles/min.**

4. The assembly is suspended in the liquid medium in a 1000 ml beaker.

5. Below the beaker there is a heating device which maintains temperature of liquid 37°C during test (37°C ± 2°C).

6. There is a separate arrangement of knobs for time setting and temperature control.

Method for Uncoated Tablets

1. Six tablets are placed in each of the 6 tubes of the basket and disc is added to each tube.

2. The beaker should be filled with water and temperature should be 37°C.

3. The machine is started.

4. The tablets pass the test if all 6 tablets have disintegrated in not more than 15 minutes. If one or two tablets fail to disintegrate, the test is repeated on 12 additional tablets. The tablet passes the test if not less than 16 of toal 18 tablets disintegrate.

Disintegration Time as per IP

1. Not more than 15 minutes for uncoated tablets.

2. One hour for coated tablets.

3. Three hours for enteric coated tablets.

18 Explain "dissolution test" for tablets as per IP 85. (S. 05)

☞ Dissolution test is done for measuring the amount of time required for a given % of the drug in a tablet to go into solution under specified conditions *in vitro*.

Dissolution Test Apparatus

It consists of following parts:

1. A cylindrical covered beaker made up of glass having 1000 ml capacity.
2. The stirring shaft is placed in the beaker which is fitted with motor at upper end. To the lower end of the shaft a basket is fixed.

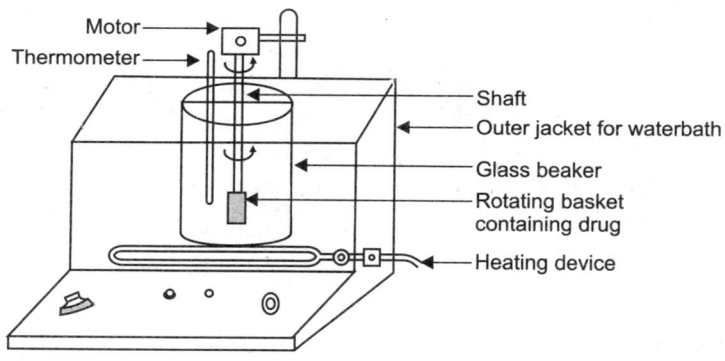

Motor

Thermometer

Shaft

Outer jacket for waterbath

Glass beaker

Rotating basket containing drug

Heating device

Dissolution test apparatus

3. A cylindrical stainless steel basket is made up of woven wire cloths having an aperture size 425 μm.
4. An electric motor which is capable of rotating the basket in the vessel have a speed of 25 to 150 rpm.
5. The beaker is fixed in the waterbath which is maintained at 37°C ± 0.5°C.

Method

1. Place 1000 ml of water which should be free from dissolved air and warm it up to 37°C.
2. Place specified number of tablets in the dry basket. Set the apparatus.
3. Start the motor and adjust rotation speed of 100 rpm and wait for 45 minutes.

4. After 45 minutes, withdraw the stated volume of solution from the vessel.
5. By analysing each sample dissolution rate is determined.

19 Define friability. Explain "friability test" for tablets.

☞ Friability

Friability means tablets may show powdering, capping, chipping, breaking into smaller pieces during normal handling, packing or transportation and produce loss in weight.

- Friability test is performed to determine ability of a tablet to with stand wear and tear during packing, handling and transportation.
- The apparatus used to perform friability test is known as **friabilator.**

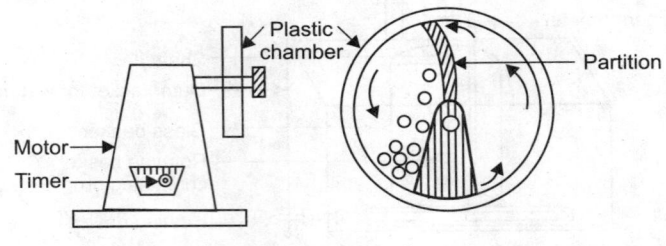

Friabilator

Apparatus

1. It consists of plastic chamber, which is divided into two parts by partition.
2. Plastic chamber is attached with a motor which revolves 25 rpm.
3. Timer is arranged at the bottom.

Method

1. Twenty tablets are weighed and placed in the plastic chamber and lid is closed.
2. The chamber is rotated for 4 minutes or 100 revolutions.
3. During each revolution the tablet falls from a distance of 6 inch.
4. After 4 minutes, the tablets are removed from the chamber and weighed.
5. The **loss in weight indicates friability.**
6. The tablets are considered to be of good quality if the loss in weight is less than 0.8%.

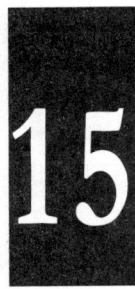

Processing of Capsule

1 Define capsule. Give merits and demerits of capsule.

☞ **Capsule (S. 97, 99, 04, 08; W. 96, 97, 98, 03)**

Capsules are a solid dosage form in which the drug substance is enclosed in a water soluble shell.

Advantages

1. It is attractive in apperance.
2. It can mask the odour, taste and colour of the medicament.
3. It is tastless.
4. It is simple to use and handling.
5. It is smooth, slipped thus easily swallowed.
6. It is economical.
7. It is available in wide range of colours and sizes.
8. Microencapsulation provides the sustained released dosage form.
9. Requires minimum additives.
10. It is physiologically inert.

Disadvantages

1. The hygroscopic drugs cannot be filled in capsules.
2. Not suitable for extremely soluble materials as they cause GIT irritation.
3. Not suitable for highly soluble compounds.
4. Aqueous or hydroalcoholic liquids cannot be enclosed in the capsules.
5. Proteolytic enzymes may interact with gelatin, thus not suitable.

2 Distinguish between 'hard gelatin and soft gelatin capsules'. (W. 04, 05)

☞

Hard gelatin capsules	Soft gelatin capsules
1. It is composed of gelatin, water and less % of plasticizer	It is composed of gelatin, water and 100% plasticizer
2. It has two parts—body and cap	It has unit body
3. It is cylindrical and hemispherical ends	It is available in different shapes like oval or spherical
4. Available in 8 standard sizes 000 to 5 (smallest)	No standard size but available in different sizes
5. Only suitable for solids	Suitable for both solids and liquids
6. Capsules are sealed after they	Filling and sealing are done are filled in a combined operation on machine
7. Hand filling and sealing is possible	Machine is required

3 Give different forms of hard gelatin capsule according to the size and capacity in milligram. (S. 98, 05; W. 98, 00)

☞

Capsule number	Approximate capacity in mg
000	950 (Largest)
00	650
0	450
1	300
2	250
3	200
4	150
5	100 (Smallest)

4 What are additives/excipients used in filling of hard gelatin capsule? (W. 96, 06)

☞1. **Diluent:** The diluent is needed when the quantity of medicament is too small, e.g. lactose, mannitol, starch.

2. **Absorbents:** These are used to absorb moisture and protect the hygroscopic substances, e.g. kaolin, magnesium oxide.

3. **Glidants:** They increase the regular flow of powder during filling, e.g. talc, magnesium stearate, calcium stearate.

4. **Antidusting agents:** Druing filling of capsule, a lot of dust comes out from the machine which may be harmful to workers. To avoid this some antidusting agents are added, e.g. inert edible oils.

5 **What are the special applications of capsule? (S. 02; W. 00, 05, 07)**

☞1. **Enteric coated capsules:** These capsules disintegrate in the intestine and not in the stomach. The shell is coated with enteric coated materials like shellac.

2. **Sustained release capsules:** These capsules produce prolonged action and reduce repeated administration of the drug. In this case coated and uncoated granules/pellets of drug are filled in a definite proportion. Uncoated granules are quickly absorbed and produce quick action while coated granules dissolve slowly thus produce prolonged drug action.

3. **Rectal capsules:** These are used for rectal administration and are substitute for rectal suppositories. These capsules contain semisolid/liquid medicament.

4. **Capsules containing ophthalmic ointment:** Nowadays ophthalmic ointments are packed in soft gelatin capsules. They contain single dose and thus they can maintain sterility of the ointment. At the time of application, the tip of capsule is punctured with sterile needle and its contents are instilled into the eye cavity and then capsule is discarded.

6 **Explain the processing/filling/manufacturing of soft gelatin capsules. (S. 99, 04, 07; W. 98, 99, 02, 03, 08)**

☞• Soft gelatin capsules are generally filled mechanically.
• The manufacturing of capsule shell and the filling of the medicament take place simultaneously.
• Rotary die machine is used for this purpose.
   1. The machine consists of two hoppers in which liquid gelatin mixture is placed.
   2. The middle hopper contains liquid medicament.
   3. There are two rotating dies which rotate in oppostie direction.

4. When fluid gelatin mixture enters the machine from the hopper, it produces two continuous ribbons.

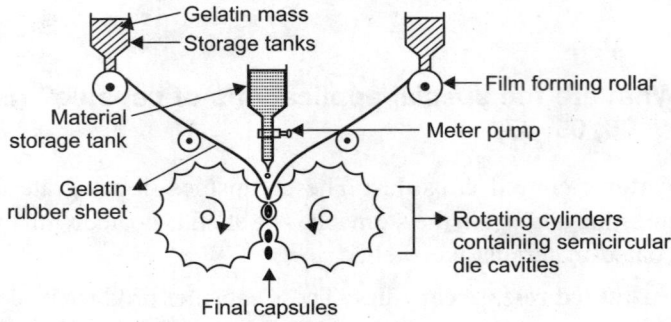

Processing of soft gelatin capsule

5. These ribbons come over the rotating dies and thus half shell of the capsule is formed.
6. In between the two cylinders the material is supplied through the pump.
7. The material exert the pressure on the gelatin sheet and press the sheet into the die cavity.
8. Due to pressure and heat two halves of the capsule are sealed.
9. The capsules formed are washed thoroughly and dried.
10. Finishing of capsule:
    – In this stage undesired matter adhered to the capsule is removed by rubbing the capsules on the piece of cloth containing inert oil.
    – Finishing provides clean and attractive apperance and lustre to the capsules.

7 Discuss processing of hard gelatin capsule. OR Discuss the operations of hand-operated hard gelatin capsule filling machine. (S. 97, 98, 01, 06, 08, 09; W. 98, 99, 01)

☞ Processing of hard gelatin capsule is divided into following steps:
1. Separation of cap from the body.
2. Filling the body.
3. Rejoining the cap and body, cleaning and polishing.
4. Packing/sealing.

Hand-operated capsule filling machines are available:

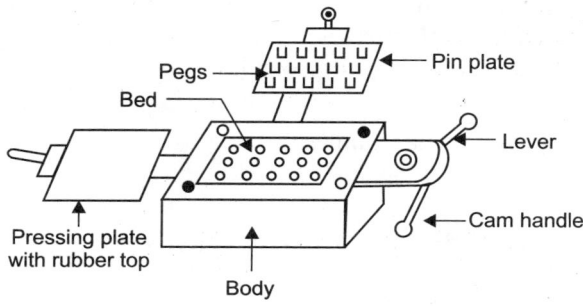

Operation

1. The empty gelatin capsules are filled in the loading tray and it is placed over the bed.
2. The cam-handle is operated to separate the caps from their bodies.
3. The powder tray is placed in a proper position and filled with an accurate quantity of powder with scrapper. The excess powder is removed.
4. The pin plate is lowered and the filled powder is pressed.
5. Then remove the pin plate and again remaining powder is filled into the bodies of capsule.
6. The powdered tray is removed after its complete filling.
7. The cap holding tray is again placed in position.
8. The plate with the rubber top is lowered and the lever is operated to lock the caps and bodies.
9. Loading tray is then removed and filled capsules are collected.
10. Cleaning of capsule is necessary to remove adhered fine dust of the material with soft cloth.
11. A cloth containing slight amount of mineral oil or a wax is used to give shining to the capsules.
12. Finally capsules are packed by using machines.

8 Give the composition of soft gelatin capsules. Give their types. (S. 98, 00, 02, 07; W. 96, 97, 00, 01)

☞ Soft gelatin capsules are also known as "soluble elastic"/"soft elastic capsule".

Composition

- Soft gelatin capsules consist of **gelatin, water** and high percentage of **plasticizer**, i.e. sorbitol or glycerin plasticizers give elastic properties to capsules.
- Preservative—methyl or propyl paraben.
- Opacifying agent—titanium dioxide.
- Flavouring agent.

Types/Shapes of Soft Gelatin Capsules

Round   Oval   Oblong   Tube   Miscellaneous

9 Enlist various evaluation tests for capsule.

☞ Capsules are evaluated for:
1. Weight variation test.
2. Content of the active ingredient in the capsule.
3. Disintegration test.
4. Dissolution test.

10 Write the packing and storage conditions of capsules. (S. 07)

☞ 1. Capsules are closed in the glass/plastic containers.
 2. Capsules are also packed in the form of blister or strip packing.

Storage

The capsules should be stored at a temperature not exceeding 30°C and in dry place.

- Storage at high humidity causes increase in moisture content and capsules stick together and at high temperature, capsule may get cracked.

Immunity and Immunological Preparations

1 **Define immunity. Classify immunity. (S. 97, 98, 04, 09; W. 00, 98, 03, 08)**

☞ **Immunity**

Immunity is the power of the body to resist effect of invasion of pathogenic microorganism in the body.

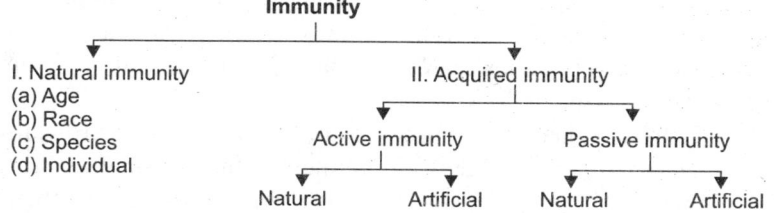

2 **Differentiate between active and passive immunity. (S. 99, 01, 09; W. 99, 04, 06, 07, 08)**

☞

Active immunity	Passive immunity
1. Antigens are injected in the human body, as a result antibodies are formed	Readymade antibodies are injected in the human body
2. It develops slowly	It develops quickly
3. It remains for longer time	It remains for short period
4. The treatment is preventive	The treatment is therapeutic

Contd.

Active immunity	Passive immunity
5. Immunological memory is present	Immunological memory is absent
6. Not useful in immunodeficient hosts	Useful to immunodeficient hosts
7. No inheritance	May be acquired from mother
8. Preparations, e.g. vaccines, toxoids	Preparations, e.g. sera

3 Define the terms. (S. 99, 00, 08; W. 98, 99, 00, 02)

☞(a) **Susceptibility:** It means unability of the body to resist infection caused by pathogenic organisms.
 (b) **Virulence:** It means ability of the organisms to produce infection.
 (c) **Antigen:** Antigens are the substances which when introduced in the body stimulate the production of antibodies.
 (d) **Antibody:** These are the substances formed in response to the stimulation of antigens in the body.
 (e) **Pathogens** are organisms capable of causing infection.
 (f) **Immunology:** The study of immunity is known as immunology.
 (g) **Carrier:** Carrier is an individual which carries and transmits pathogens but does not display himself the clinical symptoms of the disease.
 (h) **Toxoid:** When toxic properties of the toxin are destroyed by heat treatment or chemical treatment without loss of antigenic properties. Such preparations are called toxoids, e.g. diphtheria toxoid, tetanus toxoid.
 (i) **Vaccines:** Vaccines are the preparations containing antigens which stimulate the body to produce antibodies, e.g. BCG vaccine, cholera vaccine.

4 What are immunological products? Classify them. (W. 98, 03, 05)

☞ Immunological Products

These are the preparations having immunogenic properties which are used for the prevention of disease or treatment of disease and for diagnostic purposes.

Classification

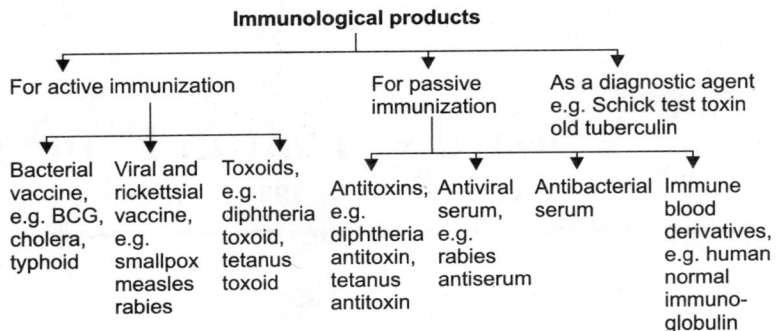

Board Question Papers
(From Summer 1995 to Summer 2017)

Summer Examination 1995
D Pharm First Year
Pharmaceutics I

Q 1. Attempt any *five* of the following:

    a. Give classification of dosage form.

    b. Why there is no single book like "World pharmacopoeia" for all the countries?

    c. What is lyophilization?

    d. What is menstrum and marc?

    e. What is extraction?

    f. What are toxoids?

    g. What is the meaning of the term "aspetic"?

Q 2. Attempt any *four* of the following:

    a. Explain principle and working of fluid energy mill.

    b. How following defects in the tablets arise and how they can be removed? Capping, picking and mottling.

    c. Give some special applications of gelatin capsules.

    d. Why injectables should not be stored in sodalime glass containers?

    e. Give uses of plastic as a material of pharmaceutical packaging.

    f. Explain mechanism of solid mixing.

Q 3. Attempt any *four* of the following:

    a. What is chemical sterilization? Which chemicals are used for this process?

    b. Explain working of Soxhlet's extractor.

    c. Why is granulation required in tablets manufacturing?

    d. Write short note on metafilter.

e. Explain importance of steam distillation in pharmacy.

f. What is the difference between antitoxins and antisenims?

Q 4. Attempt any *four* of the following:

a. Why tablets are required to evaluate for the following parameters?

    i. Friability   ii. Dissolution rate

b. What are glidants? What is their use in tablet manufacturing?

c. Explain principle and working of continuous rotary drum filters.

d. What is counter current decantation?

e. How many parts of 60%, 45% and 70% alcohol should be mixed to get 55% alcohol?

f. Give preparation of rabies vaccine IP.

Q 5. Attempt any *four* of the following:

a. Give advantages of reserved percolation.

b. What are flexible package.

c. What are the official text for rubber closures?

d. What is pasteurization?

e. Why tablets are coated?

f. What are filtration and colation? How filtration rate can be increased?

Q 6. Attempt any *four* of the following:

a. Why shaft of the propeller mixers should be deeply inserted in the container?

b. Explain spray drying with its merits and demerits.

c. What is multiple maceration? How volume of menstium required for double and triple maceration is calculated?

d. Differentiate between mixing and homogenisation.

e. How soft gelatin capsules are manufactured?

f. Convert the following into the common metric system:

    i. 1 ounce   v. 1 pint

    ii. 1 grain   vi. 1 quart

    iii. 1 minim   vii. 1 pound

    iv. 1 teaspoonful

Winter Examination 1995
D Pharm First Year
Pharmaceutics I

Q 1. Attempt any *five* of the following:

a. Define dose and dosage form.

b. What are pharmacopoeias and why they are needed?

   c. Differentiate between sterilization and disinfection.
   d. What do you mean by aseptic techniques?
   e. What is immunity?
   f. What is difference between purified water and water for injection?
   g. Give pharmaceutical importance of size reduction.

Q 2. Attempt any *four* of the following:
   a. Explain construction and working of ball mill.
   b. Explain various types of mixtures with their relative stability.
   c. What are advantages and disadvantages of rubber as a material for closure?
   d. What is size separation, define coarse, moderately coarse and very fine powders?
   e. Explain gaseous sterilization.
   f. Explain reserved percolation.

Q 3. Attempt any *four* of the following:
   a. Why tablets are most popular dosage forms.
   b. What are the advantages and disadvantages of implants.
   c. Explain principle and construction of cyclone separator.
   d. What are filter aids?
   e. What are vaccines? How BCG vaccine is prepared?
   f. What are surgical ligatures and sutures?

Q 4. Attempt any *four* of the following:
   a. Differentiate between hard gelatin and soft gelatin capsules.
   b. Explain principle and working of an autoclave.
   c. Explain homogenization.
   d. What are advantages and disadvantages of filter press?
   e. Explain principle of extraction of organized drugs.
   f. Explain various factors affecting evaporation.

Q 5. Attempt any *four* of the following:
   a. Explain various steps involved in sugar coating of tablet.
   b. Explain method of preparation of water for injection.
   c. How many parts of 60%, 48%, 40% and 35% alcohol should be mixed to get 50% alcohol?
   d. What is official test for bacteria proof filters? Name the commonly used filters for the sterilization.
   e. What are plasticizers and what is their role in preparation of soft gelatin capsules.
   f. Define lyophilization.

Q 6. Which instrument you will suggest for the following operation? Explain giving reasons (any *four*).

    a. For size reduction of wet filter press cake.

    b. For mixing of an ointment ingredients.

    c. For filtration of 10% sucrose solution.

    d. For extraction of a drug of high therapeutic value

    e. For drying of a thermolabile material.

    f. For making sterile eyedrops.

Winter Examination 1996
D Pharm First Year
Pharmaceutics I

Q 1. Solve any *five* of the following:

    a. How will you prepare 1 quart of 1 in 400 solution of potassium permanganate?

    b. Define "drug" and "dosage form".

    c. Classify additives used in formulation of dosage form.

    d. What are the basic objectives of publication of pharmacopoeias?

    e. Define "metrology". Name the various systems of weights and measures followed in pharmacy.

    f. What are the objectives of mixing?

    g. Define "filtration" and "clarification" "slurry" and "filter cake".

Q 2. Attempt any *four* of the following:

    a. What are the natural defence mechanisms to which immunity is due? Name the various types of immunological preparations used commonly.

    b. How will you prepare "diphtheria antitoxin"?

    c. Differentiate between "hard and soft gelatin capsules".

    d. Name the various processes used under "moist heat sterilization". Explain the working of "autoclave".

    e. Define "drying". Give the construction and working a vacuum dryer.

    f. What is "vacuum distillation"? What is its principle? Draw a labelled sketch of small scale vacuum distillation assembly.

Q 3. Attempt any *four* of the following:

    a. What is the theory of filtration process? Explain the working of sintered glass filter.

    b. What are the mechanism of powder mixing? Explain the working of double cone blender.

c. How will you separate the particles of different sizes from a suspension? Explain the working of cyclone separator.

d. Name the various materials used in pharmaceutical packaging. Give details about advantages and drawbacks of glass as a container.

e. Name the factors affecting size reduction. Give the construction and working of "ball mill".

f. Explain the principle of soxhlation. Explain the working of "Soxhlet's extractor".

Q 4. Solve any *four* of the following:

a. What is aseptic technique? What are the various sources of contamination? Where is this technique followed? Give a diagram of aseptic chamber.

b. Define "toxin" and "toxoid". Explain about various toxin containing preparations used for diagnostic purpose.

c. What are various additives used in capsule formulation? What are special applications of capsules?

d. Name and explain the various defects in tableting.

e. What is "digestion"? Explain the process by which tincture from crude drug can be obtained.

f. What is the importance of rubber as material for closure? Name the various tests that rubber has to comply with.

Q 5. Solve any *four* of the following:

a. What is "alligation". In what proportions 40, 20 and 10 percent ointments be mixed to get 25% ointment?

b. Write a note on "form giver and form stabilizer" in a dosage form.

c. Discuss about the various developments that took place before the publication of first Indian pharmacopoeia.

d. What are advantages of granules over fine powder in tableting?

e. Name the various official standards specified for tablets. Give details of "dissolation rate test".

f. Name the commonly used gases for sterilisation. Give details about ethylene oxide.

Q 6. Solve any *four* of the following:

a. What is viral vaccine? How shall you prepare smallpox vaccine using eggs?

b. What are the various advantages of capsules?

c. What are the qualities of a good tablet? What do you mean by "enteric coated tablet"?

d. Explain about sterilisation by radiation.

e. Explain the construction and working of compartment dryer.

f. Explain the various factors affecting rate of filtration.

Summer Examination 1997
D Pharm First Year
Pharmaceutics I

Q 1. Answer any *five* of the following:

  a. What do you mean by active immunity and passive immunity?
  b. Give reasons for coating the tablets.
  c. What is sterilization by radiation? Give its importance.
  d. Give any two advantages and disadvantages of evaporating pan.
  e. What is maceration? Describe in short.
  f. Give any four factors affecting rate of filtration or evaporation.
  g. What is sieve number? State official grades of powders.

Q 2. Answer any *four* of the following:

  a. Give merits and demerits of solid dosage forms.
  b. Describe construction and working of hammer mill.
  c. What is percolation? Give various stages involved in carrying out official percolation process.
  d. Describe construction and working of fluidised bed dryer.
  e. Classify the tablets depending on their route of administration.
  f. Describe construction and working of hand-operated capsule filling machine.

Q 3. Answer any *four* of the following:

  a. Define pharmacopoeia. Write a note on history of Indian pharmacopoeia.
  b. Give importance of size reduction in pharmacy.
  c. What is ayurvedic medicine? Define following with at least one example of each:
      i. Avaleha   iii. Bhasma
      ii. Gutika
  d. Describe the structure of vacuum oven. Give its application in pharmacy.
  e. Name the types of tablet excipients. Define following with at least one example of each:
      i. Diluent   ii. Lubricant
  f. Define sterilization. Classify methods of sterilization.

Q 4. Answer any *four* of the following:

  a. A pharmacist has three lots of ichthamol ointment containing 30%, 18% and 12% of ichthamol respectively. In what proportion should these be mixed to obtain an ointment containing 15% of ichthamol?

    b. What are various methods of size separation? Describe construction of cyclone separator.

    c. What is lyophilization? Give its application in pharmaceutical industry.

    d. Describe in brief sterilization by filtration with its advantages and disadvantages.

    e. What are the problems involved in tablet manufacture? What is binding and chipping?

    f. What is aerosol packaging and give any two advantages and disadvantages.

Q 5. Answer any *four* of the following:

    a. Define isotonic solution. Give the effects of injecting hypotonic solutions. Give general principles of adjustment of tonicity.

    b. Describe various factors affecting mixing.

    c. When distillation under reduced pressure is essential? Draw a well labelled diagram of vacuum still.

    d. Define immunity and immunisation. Classify immunity.

    e. What is sterile water for injection? How is it prepared?

    f. Define filter medium and filter aid with suitable examples.

Q 6. Answer any *four* of the following:

    a. What is closure? Give various types of closure. Which material is used for making closures?

    b. Name the equipments used for mixing solids with liquids. Describe planetary mixer.

    c. Define evaporation. Give any four factors affecting evaporation.

    d. Differentiate between antitoxins and antisera.

    e. Enlist the quality control tests for tablets as per IP 85. Describe test for friability.

    f. Give advantages and disadvantages of capsules.

Summer Examination 1998
D Pharm First Year
Pharmaceutics I

Q 1. Answer any *five* of the following:

    a. What are paratonic solutions? What are the effects of injecting hypertonic solutions?

    b. Define container. Name any two materials widely used for containers.

   c. Give any four advantages of ball mill.

   d. Give any four factors affecting mixing.

   e. Define with one example each:
      i. Arka   ii. Lepa

   f. Describe in brief capping of tablet and mottling of tablet.

   g. Give any two advantages and disadvantages of sterilization by filtration.

Q 2. Answer any *four* of the following:

   a. Broadly classify pharmaceutical dosage forms. Give any two merits and demerits of injectables.

   b. Give application of size reduction in pharmacy.

   c. Describe working of a Soxhlet's apparatus with neat labelled diagram.

   d. Describe the construction and working of a fluidised bed dryer with diagram.

   e. Give any four advantages and disadvantages of tablets.

   f. What is pharmacopoeia? Write a short note on Indian pharmacopoeia.

Q 3. Answer any *four* of the following:

   a. How many parts of 90%, 80%, 60% and 40% alcohol should be mixed so as to obtain alcohol of 70% strength?

   b. Describe construction and working of cyclone separator.

   c. What is lyophilization? Describe process of freeze drying with its applications.

   d. Define sterilization. Classify methods of sterilization.

   e. Mention the steps involved in preparation of dry granulation. Give its advantages over fine powder.

   f. What is the principle of test for sterility? How test for sterility is carried out?

Q 4. Answer any *four* of the following:

   a. Give any four advantages and disadvantages of glass when it is used as material for container.

   b. Name various equipment used for mixing of powders. Describe any one of them.

   c. Enumerate the factors affecting evaporation.

   d. Describe how viral and rickettial vaccines are prepared? How are they stored?

   e. Mention various quality control tests for tablets. Describe the apparatus used for disintegration test.

   f. Define capsule. Describe various types of capsules.

Q 5. Answer any *four* of the following:

a. What is tamper resistant packaging? Classify it and give advantages of any one of them.

b. What are the properties of an ideal filter medium?

c. Describe the fractional distillation with a diagram of fractionating column.

d. What is immunity? Classify immunity.

e. Describe the construction and application of the apparatus used for moist heat sterilization.

f. What is drying? Write a note on theory of drying.

Q 6. Answer any *four* of the following:

a. Give requirements of an ideal diluent for tablet.

b. Describe construction and working of a filter press with a diagram.

c. What is mixing? Describe factors affecting mixing.

d. Describe construction and working of evaporating pan with diagram.

e. Define with example:
   i. Asava and Arishta   ii. Anjana

f. Describe the construction and working of hand-operated capsule filling machine.

Winter Examination 1998
D Pharm First Year
Pharmaceutics I

Q 1. Attempt any *five* of the following:

a. Define "drug" and "additives".

b. Prepare 4 oz of a solution so that 1 tablespoonful to 1 quart makes 1 in 500 solution.

c. Name the various materials used for containers. What is well closed container?

d. Why is lime soda glass not used for storage of parenteral products?

e. Name at least four factors affecting size reduction.

f. What is elutriation process?

g. What are advantages of filter press?

Q 2. Solve any *four* of the following:

a. Explain the construction and working of metafilter.

b. What is percolation? Name the stages involved in it. What is d/p ratio in extracts?

c. What are the various new drug delivery systems? What are advantages of sustained action dosage form?

d. What are salient features of III edition of IP? When was II edition published?

e. What are the qualities which an ideal container should possess?

f. Explain the construction and working of disintegrator.

Q 3. Solve any *four* of the following:

a. Name and explain various types of mixtures.

b. Explain the construction and working of triple roller mill or colloid mill.

c. Define filtration and clarification. Enumerate advantages of sintered glass filter.

d. Explain the construction and working of evaporating pan or evaporating still.

e. Name various ayurvedic dosage forms with suitable examples.

f. What is "dry heat sterilisation"? Explain the working of hot air oven.

Q 4. Attempt any *four* of the following:

a. What are various stages involved in sterilisation of surgical dressings?

b. Define "capsules". Name the various additives used in capsule formulation.

c. What is "slugging"? What are the advantages of granules in tablet compression?

d. What are the various additives used in mixture formulation? Explain with examples.

e. How are hard gelatin capsules filled and sealed using capsule filling machine (hand-operated)?

f. Find the concentration of sodium chloride required to make 1.5% solution of cocaine hydrochloride isotonic with blood plasma. (Freezing point of 1% w/v of concentrated HCl is – 0.09°C. Freezing point of 1% w/v of sodium chloride is – 0.576°C).

Q 5. Solve any *four* of the following:

a. Define "immunity". Classify it. Explain natural immunity.

b. What do you understand by "immunological preparation"? Name the various types of such preparations. What are toxin and toxoid?

c. Explain the various properties of "hard gelatin capsules".

d. What are advantages of coating? Explain sugar coating.

e. Name the various standards for compressed tablets. Explain the "dissolution test".

f. How is "test for sterility" performed?

Summer Examination 1999
D Pharm First Year
Pharmaceutics I

Q 1. Answer any *five* of the following:

a. What do you mean by immunisation?

b. Which are the ideal characteristics of tablets? Mention any four.

c. What is aseptic processing? Which precautions should be taken during aseptic processing?

d. Give the principle of distillation under reduced pressure.

e. What is maceration? Describe in short.

f. What is packaging and package?

g. State the importance of size reduction in emulsion and suspension.

Q 2. Answer any *four* of the following:

a. Give any four merits and demerits of liquid dosage forms.

b. Describe construction and operation of a fluid energy mill with a diagram.

c. What is imbibition? Give reasons for imbibition during percolation.

d. Describe structure, principle and application of tray dryer.

e. Classify the tablets on the basis of their routes of administration and function.

f. Define pharmaceutical aid. Mention any two types of pharmaceutical aid with one example of each.

Q 3. Answer any *four* of the following:

a. Name various excipients used in tablet formulation with at least one example of each.

b. What is sieve number? State official grades of powders.

c. Differentiate between maceration and percolation.

d. Describe vacuum oven. Give its advantages.

e. How many editions of Indian pharmacopoeia are published so far? What are the salient features of IP 85?

f. Define metrology. In what proportion should 15%, 12% and 4% sulphur ointment be mixed in order to obtain a mixture of 8% ointment?

Q 4. Answer any *four* of the following:

   a. Give any three advantages and disadvantages of plastic as a material for container.

   b. What are the mechanisms of mixing? Give various factors affecting mixing.

   c. Classify the ayurvedic dosage forms on the basis of physical form with one example of each.

   d. Name various methods of sterilization. Describe in short sterilization by heating with bactericide.

   e. Describe direct compression of tablet with its advantages and disadvantages.

   f. Describe the construction, operation and application of Silverson mixer homogeniser.

Q 5. Answer any *four* of the following:

   a. What do you mean by aerosol? Give its advantages and disadvantages.

   b. What are filtration and clarification? Give any three factors affecting rate of filtration.

   c. Describe structure and working of evaporating pan with diagram.

   d. Give advantages and disadvantages of sterilization by filtration. Name any two filter units used for the purpose of filtrations.

   e. Differentiate between active immunity and passive immunity with one official immunological preparation of each.

   f. How are soft gelatin capsules prepared and filled?

Q 6. Answer any *four* of the following:

   a. Describe in short metafilter with a diagram and give its application.

   b. What is pyrogen? How is sterile water for injection prepared?

   c. Give method of preparation and storage conditions for smallpox vaccine.

   d. Why tablets should be coated? Describe in short enteric coating.

   e. Describe the process of steam distillation and equipment used for the same.

   f. Give advantages and disadvantages of capsules.

Summer Examination 2000
D Pharm First Year
Pharmaceutics I

Q 1. Answer any *five* of the following:

   a. Define:

      i. Syrups   ii. Elixirs

    b. What are the advantages of suppository dosage form?

    c. How much quantity of dextrose will be required for making 500 ml solution of dextrose isotonic with blood plasma, molecular weight of dextrose is 180 and it is nonionising.

    d. What are the ideal properties of filter media?

    e. Name the method for sterilisation of:

        i. An injection containing thermolabile drug

        ii. Surgical hand gloves

        iii. Aseptic cabinet

        iv. Rubber closures

Q 2. Answer any *four* of the following:

    a. What are the official standards for powder size?

    b. Describe the construction, working and advantages of fluid energy mill.

    c. What are the desirable characteristics of containers used in packaging of pharmaceuticals?

    d. How will you prepare 300 ml of potassium permanganate solution such that when 20 ml of this diluted with water to 200 ml will give 1 in 500 solution of potassium permanganate. Label—use the dilute solution having the strength 1 in 500 for washing the gums and teeth.

    e. Write a note on implants.

Q 3. Answer any *four* of the following:

    a. Describe the history of Indian pharmacopoeia.

    b. Name the principles of size reduction and mention the mills based on those principles.

    c. What is sieving? How does IP define No. 10 sieve?

    d. Write a note on powder mixing.

    e. Discuss in brief different types of filter media used in pharmacy.

Q 4. Answer any *four* of the following:

    a. Discuss briefly the role of positive pressure air lock system and ultraviolet lamps in sterile area.

    b. Write a note on water for injection IP.

    c. What are the applications of distillation under reduced pressure?

    d. Explain evaporating still. What are its advantages and disadvantages?

    e. What are the requirements of satisfactory tablets?

Q 5. Answer any *four* of the following:

    a. Explain the need of granulation in the processing of tablets.

    b. Differentiate between hard gelatin and soft gelatin capsule.

c. Define immunity. What is the difference between antigen and serum?

d. What are toxoids? Give two examples of it. Discuss general methods of preparation of toxoids.

e. Explain why unorganised drugs are usually not extracted by percolation and marc is never pressed after extraction of unorganised drugs.

Q 6. Answer any *four* of the following:

a. What are the pharmaceutical applications of freeze drying? What are the advantages of freeze drying?

b. Describe in brief process of percolation.

c. Write in brief preparation of smallpox vaccine using animal.

d. What is the purpose of enteric coating? Give three examples each of enteric film, former material and solvents used in enteric coating.

e. Mention different official and nonofficial tests for evaluation of tablets. Discuss disintegration test for uncoated tablets.

Winter Examination 2000
D Pharm First Year
Pharmaceutics I

Q 1. Attempt any *five* of the following:

a. Define pharmacopoeia and official substance.

b. What is targeted drug delivery system? Which different types does it include?

c. Define "imperial standard pound" and "litre".

d. Name various types of closures used.

e. What are the objectives of size reduction?

f. What are functions and properties of "filter aids".

g. Explain the working of hand homogeniser.

h. What are special applications of capsules?

Q 2. Answer any *four* of the following:

a. Define "capsule". What is the composition of hard and soft gelatin capsule shell?

b. Define "immunity" and "susceptibility". Classify immunity. What are antigenic preparations?

c. What are the various additives used in tablet formulation. Explain with examples.

d. What is sterilisation? How sterilisation differs from disinfection? Name two disinfectants.

   e. Why is it necessary to coat the tablets? Name the different methods used for it. Explain film coating.

   f. Where is freeze drying used? Explain the theory and stages involved in freeze drying.

Q 3. Attempt any *four* of the following:

   a. What is "microencapsulation"? What are its advantages?

   b. Name the various heat processes used in pharmacy. Explain the importance of steam as a source of heat.

   c. What is evaporation. Describe factors affecting rate of evaporation.

   d. What are the advantages of "reserve percolation process"? Explain the process.

   e. Give a broad classification of various dosage forms. Give detailed classification of solid dosage form.

Q 4. Attempt any *four* of the following:

   a. What is isotonic solution? What is the effect of injecting hypotonic solution.

      Find the proportion of sodium chloride required to make 1% solution of cocaine hydrochloride isotonic.

      (Freezing point of 1% NaCl is $-0.576°C$ and that of cocaine HCl is $-0.09°C$).

   b. Name the various ayurvedic dosage forms. Define "Avaledha" "Kupipakva Rasayan".

   c. What is "monograph"? What are specifications given about "solubiltiy" in the monograph?

   d. Name the various packaging materials used in pharmacy. What is "aerosol package"? Give the advantage of it.

   e. Explain the construction and working of a size reduction mill working on the principle of "impact".

   f. What is size separation? What do you understand by "sieve no. 20"? Which are official grades for the powders?

Q 5. Attempt any *four* of the following:

   a. Define "filter medium". What are its character and functions? Quote the suitable examples.

   b. Define "compressed tablet". Name the various processes used to prepare it. Explain moist granulation process.

   c. What is the difference between "purified water" "water for injection" and "sterile water for injection"? How shall you prepare distilled water continuously.

   d. What is maceration? Name the types of products prepared by using it.

Differentiate between the process used for organised and unorganised drugs.

e. Name the various types of preparations used in active immunisation. How shall you prepare BCG vaccine in freeze dried form?

f. Explain the construction and working of "fluidised bed dryer" or double cone mixer.

Q 6. Attempt any *four* of the following:

a. Explain about the points to be considered while formulating a dosage form.

b. What are the characteristic features of third edition of IP? When was it published?

c. Write a note on "plastic" as packaging medium.

d. Explain the construction and working of "agitator mixer".

e. What is fractional distillation? Draw fractionating distillation assembly.
What is the function of "fractionating column"?

f. Write a note on "bacterial filtration sterilization"?

Summer Examination 2001
D Pharm First Year
Pharmaceutics I

Q 1. Answer any *five* of the following:

a. Name various mechanisms of size reduction along with different mills based on each of them.

b. Differentiate between active and passive immunity.

c. What is the principle behind distillation under reduced pressure?

d. Define 'churna' and 'bhasma'.

e. What is sterilisation? Mention various methods of sterilisation.

f. Why is enteric coating given to some tablets?

g. Give the metric equivalents of the following:
   i. One pint   iii. 15 grains
   ii. One tablespoonful

Q 2. Answer any *four* of the following:

a. Describe in brief dry granulation method.

b. Give classification of tablets. Only mention official and nonofficial standards for tablets.

c. Describe in brief processing of 'hard gelatin capsules'.

d. Describe in brief test for weight variation in the tablets.

e. Write note on sedimentation method of size separation.

f. Explain microencapsulation technique for tablet coating.

Q 3. Answer any *four* of the following:

a. What precautions will you take during aseptic working?

b. Discuss sterilisation by heating with bactericides.

c. What are dosage forms? How are they classified?

d. Describe the history of Indian pharmacopoeia.

e. Fill in the blanks:
  i. 1 drop = _____ ml.
  ii. 1 gallon = _____ fl ounces.
  iii. _____ scruple = 1 grain.
  iv. _____ minims = 1 fl drachm.
  v. 1 ounce = _____ grains.

f. Send 100 ml of a solution of potassium permanganate of which one part diluted with seven parts of water makes a 1 in 8000 solution.

Q 4. Answer any *four* of the following:

a. Define container and closure. State different types of containers.

b. Describe aerosol packaging, with its advantages and disadvantages.

c. Describe the principle, construction and working of disintegrator.

d. Write note on hand homogeniser.

e. What are the different quality control tests for hard gelatin capsules?

f. What is filtration? Describe briefly various filter medias.

Q 5. Answer any *four* of the following:

a. Define evaporation. Enlist the factors affecting rate of evaporation.

b. What is fractional distillation? Give its applications in pharmacy.

c. Explain principle of freeze drying. Describe the process in brief.

d. What is reserved perculation process? How is it carried out?

e. Differentiate between natural and naturally acquired immunity.

f. Find out the weight of sodium sulfate required for 100 ml of solution isotonic with blood serum.
  Given: Mol weight of sodium sulfate = 322
        Mol weight of sodium chloride = 58.5

Q 6. Answer any *four* of the following:

a. 100 g of a powder containing 8% of medicament is to be prepared from a lot of a powders containing 12% medicament and 6% medicament. Calculate the respective quantities of powders with 20% medicament and 6% medicament.

b. Explain grading of solids as per IP.

c. Explain principle and construction of cyclone separator.

d. What are vaccines? How BCG vaccine is prepared?

e. Explain spray drying with its merits and demerits.

f. Write short notes on any two of the following:

    i. National formulary

    ii. Implants

    iii. Moist heat sterilisation

Winter Examination 2001
D Pharm First Year
Pharmaceutics I

Q 1. Solve any *ten* of the following:

a. Define 'tablet'. Mention any four types of tablets.

b. Give the advantages of triple maceration over simple maceration.

c. Explain in short the term "exosmosis".

d. Enlist the steps involved in the process of extraction.

e. Give the advantages of autoclaving.

f. Give the meaning of stock vaccines.

g. Define "toxoids" How they differ from antitoxins.

h. Define 'infusion' and 'decoction'.

i. Write a note on rubber as material for closures.

j. Give any two advantages and disadvantages of metafilter.

k. Give any four examples of filter aids.

l. Enlist any four objectives of size reduction in pharmaceuticals.

m. Define 'evaporation' and give its application.

n. Name the liquids which are filled in soft gelatin capsules.

Q 2. Solve any *four* of the following:

a. Discuss in brief role of levigating agent with suitable examples.

b. Discuss in brief construction and working of ball mill.

c. Discuss in brief process of filling of capsules.

d. How many grams of sodium chloride are required to prepare 2 litres of 1 in 2000 solution.

e. Why prefiltration treatment is required? Give names of any two methods used for the same.

f. Classify the ayurvedic doses forms with suitable examples for each.

Q 3. Solve any *four* of the following:

a. Give the preparation of *vaccinium varialae*, along with its dose and use.

b. Define 'percolation'. Discuss in brief the process of percolation stepwise.

c. Discuss in brief gaseous sterilization with two applications of it.

d. Discuss in short weight variation test for tablets.

e. What do you mean by isotonic and paratonic solutions.

f. What will be the percentage of alcohol in a mixture obtained by mixing 5 litres of 25%, 1 litre of 50% and 2 litres of 95% alcohol?

Q 4. Solve any *four* of the following:

a. Convert into metric equivalents.
   i. One fluid dracum
   ii. One minim
   iii. One tablespoonful
   iv. One gallon
   v. One drop
   vi. One scruple

b. Discuss in brief working and construction of fluid energy mill.

c. Draw well labelled diagram for aerosol packaging with its application.

d. Mention any four features of container and closures.

e. How will you prepare 10% salicylic acid ointment from 40% salicylic acid ointment.

f. Give the working of triple roller mill and give its applications.

Q 5. Solve any *four* of the following:

a. Mention types of coating and discuss in brief enteric coating for tablets.

b. State in brief how the aerosols are classified on the basis of particle size.

c. Discuss in brief sintered glass filter with its applications.

d. Enlist the official tests for standardization of tablets with note on dissolution test.

e. Define 'distillation'. How it differs from evaporation.

f. How the hard gelatin capsules differ from soft gelatin capsules.

Q 6. Solve any *four* of the following:

a. Define "menstrum and marc", give the ideal qualities of menstrum.

b. Discuss in brief principle involved in vacuum-drying.

c. Enlist the official standards for powder.

d. Draw well labelled diagram for steam-distillation.

e. Discuss in brief method used for preparation of purified water IP.

f. Discuss in brief filter-candles and give their two applications.

Summer Examination 2002
D Pharm First Year
Pharmaceutics I

Q 1. Solve any _ten_ of the following:

a. Enlist the galenicals used in medical profession.

b. Define—"extraction".

c. Give any four precautions to be taken for aseptic work.

d. Mention any four main applications of gamma radiation sterilization.

e. Define—'sterilization' and 'disinfection'.

f. Name any four official vaccines.

g. How many grams of dextrose will be required to prepare 10 litres of 2.5% solution of dextrose.

h. Give any two advantages and disadvantages of filter press.

i. Name any four methods of filtration used for sterilization.

j. Enlist the objectives of mixing and homogenisation.

k. Define—'pharmaceutical container' and 'closure'.

l. Mention any four tablet excipients with one example of each.

m. Convert the following into metric equivalents.

    i. One pint   iii. One ounce

    ii. One dracum   iv. Quart

n. How is the camphor to be triturated to get the powder camphor?

Q 2. Solve any _four_ of the following:

a. Define—maceration and discuss in brief double maceration process.

b. Discuss in brief sterilization by radiation.

c. Give the preparation of Staphylococcus toxoid IP, condition of label; storage and use.

d. Calculate the amount of $KMnO_4$ required to prepare five liters of 1 in 4000 solution.

e. Draw neat and well labelled diagram of plate and frame, filter press.

f. What is pharmacopoeia? Give the history of Indian pharmacopoeia.

Q 3. Solve any _four_ of the following:

a. Discuss in brief working and principle of fluid energy mill.

b. Draw well labelled diagram for aerosol packaging.

c. Give the advantages of tablets over parenterals. Give disadvantages of tablets.

d. Discuss in brief construction and working of silverson mixture homogenizer with its advantages.

    e. How do the hard gelatin capsules differ from soft gelatin capsules?

    f. Give the principle of sedimentation method of size separation?

Q 4. Solve any *four* of the following:

    a. Mention the official tests for standardization of tablets. Discuss in short dissolution test.

    b. Translate to English:
        i. Singuli
       ii. Omani mane
      iii. Tabella
      iv. Collyrium
       v. Dispensa
      vi. Antijenta culum

    c. Mention the official tests for rubber closures and discuss any one of them.

    d. Draw well labelled diagram of "fluid energy mill".

    e. Discuss in brief sintered glass filter with its advantages (any *two*).

    f. Mention methods used in clarification and name any two clarifying agents.

Q 5. Solve any *four* of the following:

    a. Define—'distillation'. How does it differ from evaporation?

    b. Mention the mechanisms by which heat transfer takes place and explain it in brief.

    c. Give special applications of capsules.

    d. Give the importance of drying in pharmaceuticals and give the advantage of fluidized bed dryer.

    e. Mention the factors on which the efficiency of drug extraction depends.

    f. Why are granules preferred for preparation of tablets over the powder.

Q 6. Solve any *four* of the following:

    a. Define—'menstrum and marc'. State ideal qualities of menstrum.

    b. Discuss in brief process of fractional distillation and give its two applications.

    c. Define—'boiling point', state in brief how the pressure affects the boiling point of any liquid.

    d. Draw labelled diagram of filtration assembly using candle filter.

    e. How will you prepare 55% ointment from 90%; 70%; 40% and 30% stock ointment using alligation method.

    f. Enlist various Ayurvedic dosage forms.

Winter Examination 2002
D Pharm First Year
Pharmaceutics I

Q 1. Answer any *five* of the following:

a. What is sieve number? State official grades of powders.

b. Name the methods for the sterilisation of:
   - i. Surgical handgloves
   - ii. Aseptic cabinet
   - iii. Surgical powder
   - iv. An apron

c. Define the terms "antigens" and " antibodies".

d. Give any four factors and their effect on the rate of filtration.

e. What is pharmacopoeia?

f. Explain the terms "sterility" and "sterilisation".

g. What is imbibition? State its importance in percolation.

Q 2. Answer any *four* of the following:

a. Give principle, construction and working of ball mill.

b. Define mixing and homogenisation. Give the types of mixtures.

c. Classify the equipments used for liquid mixing. Describe any one of them.

d. Write short note on cyclone separator.

e. Explain process of levigation.

f. Draw a well labelled diagram of silverson homogeniser. Give its advantages and disadvantages.

Q 3. Answer any *four* of the following:

a. Explain the theory of filtration.

b. Name the different filtering devices. Describe meta-filter.

c. Define extraction. Describe the different methods of extraction.

d. What are the properties of ideal solvent used for extraction process.

e. Describe multiple maceration process.

f. Draw a well labelled diagram of Soxhlet's apparatus. Explain continuous hot extraction method.

Q 4. Answer any *four* of the following:

a. Define ayurvedic drugs. How are ayurvedic dosage forms classified? Give their examples.

b. Give the salient feature of the third edition of Indian Pharmacopoeia (IP 1985).

c. Define efflorescence and exsiccation.

d. Differentiate between evaporation and distillation.

e. Give the construction, working, advantages and disadvantages of evaporating still.

f. Convert the following into the common metric system.

   i. One ounce   iv. One teaspoonful

   ii. One pound   v. One pint

   iii. One grain

Q 5. Answer any *four* of the following:

a. Write different mechanisms of heat transfer and explain it with examples.

b. How can water for injection IP be prepared?

c. Give the principle and application of vacuum distillation.

d. Give the construction, working, advantages and disadvantages of 'fluidized bed dryer'.

e. What is chemical sterilisation? Name four chemicals which are used in this process.

f. How many parts of 60%, 48%, 40% and 35% alcohols should be mixed to get 50% alcohol?

Q 6. Answer any *four* of the following:

a. Explain the necessity of granulation in procession of compressed tablets. Name the methods of granulation.

b. Comment on the different tablets excipients.

c. Differentiate between hard gelatin capsules and soft gelatin capsules.

d. Give method of preparation of "smallpox" vaccine from eggs.

e. Define closures. Give brief account of different types of closures.

f. Comment on "Novel Drug Delivery System".

Summer Examination 2003
D Pharm First Year
Pharmaceutics I

Q 1. Solve any *ten* of the following:

a. Define—organised and unorganised crude drugs with suitable examples.

b. Define—'imbibition'.

c. Give the synonym of diphtheria antitoxin IP.

d. Differentiate between infusion and decoction.

e. Differentiate between compressed tablets and solution tablets.

f. How are the sintered glass filters to be washed?

g. Enlist the factors which affect the size reduction.

h. Give the principle of evaporation.

i. Give any four applications of evaporation.

j. In what respect water for injection differ from distilled water?

k. What is double cone mixer? Give its applications.

l. Define levigation with suitable example of levigating agents.

m. Give the name of equipment used for small scale comminution in a laboratory.

n. Name the mill which works on the principle of combined impact and attrition.

Q 2. Solve any *four* of the following:

a. Discuss in brief dissolution test for tablets and give its importance.

b. Calculate the volume required to prepare solution of 10% of 200 ml from solution of 30% hydrochloric acid.

c. What is Indian pharmacopoeia? Give its history in brief.

d. State the official standards for powders.

e. Discuss in brief mechanism involved in liquid mixing.

f. Draw well labelled diagram for hot continuous extraction and give the name of the apparatus used for it.

Q 3. Solve any *four* of the following:

a. State where the gaseous sterilization is possible. Mention the names of gases used.

b. Discuss in brief procedure for preparation of BCG, its storage, dose and use.

c. Enlist the antitoxins under IP.

d. Explain the term filter aid; give the names of agents used as filter aids in pharmaceuticals.

e. Give the importance of sera.

f. Convert the following into metric equivalents:

i. One fluid ounce	iv. One pint
ii. Quart	v. Gallon
iii. One dessert spoonful	vi. One minim

Q 4. Solve any *four* of the following:

a. Draw labelled diagram for evaporating pan and give its two applications.

b. Discuss in brief method used for preparation of purified water IP.

c. Discuss in brief processing of hard gelatin capsules.

d. Discuss in brief freeze drying process and give its two important applications.

e. Draw diagram of hammer mill and give its applications.

f. Mention any four features of container and closures.

Q 5. Solve any *four* of the following:

a. State why coating for tablets is required. Mention different types of coating.

b. Write a note on ayurvedic dosage forms.

c. How will you prepare 5% salicylic acid ointment from 25% salicylic acid ointment by using alligation method?

d. Give the principle of cyclone separator with its application.

e. Discuss in brief: How the aerosols are classified on the basis of particle size.

f. Give any three advantages and disadvantages of fluid energy mill.

Q 6. Solve any *four* of the following:

a. State the methods of granulation of tablets and discuss in brief any one of them.

b. Draw neat and well labelled diagram of plate and frame filter press.

c. Write a note on 'sterilisation by radiation'.

d. Define "percolation". Give the advantages of reserve percolation process.

e. Give the principle of "distillation under reduced pressure" and give its application.

f. Calculate the amount of $KMnO_4$ required to prepare 3 litres of 1 in 2000 solution.

Winter Examination 2003
D Pharm First Year
Pharmaceutics I

Q 1. Solve any *ten* of the following:

a. What are the factors which affect size reduction?

b. Differentiate between sustained release and controlled release dosage form.

c. Define alligation method. Give its application.

d. What are the requirements for ideal filter media?

e. Give various defects in tablet manufacturing.

f. Differentiate between spirit and tincture.

g. Give principle of extraction of an organised drug.

h. Give principle of sterilization with moist heat.

i. What is enteric coating? Give its significance.

j. Give various precautions for safe and effective handling of sterilization equipment.

k. Dispense 150 ml of eyewash containing 1% boric acid.

l. Define isotonic solution. What will be the effect if hypertonic solution is injected?

m. What are advantages of capsules over tablets?

n. What are differences between purified water and water for injection IP.

Q 2. Solve any _four_ of the following:

a. Define vaccines. Explain the process of preparation of rickettsial vaccines.

b. Give three merits and demerits of glass as a material used for container.

c. Enlist various official quality control tests for tablets. Describe apparatus used for disintegration test.

d. Differentiate between evaporation, distillation and drying.

e. Explain the construction and working of triple roller mill.

f. What are galenicals? Give methods of preparation of galenical.

Q 3. Solve any _four_ of the following:

a. Explain processing of soft gelatin capsule.

b. How will you carry out extraction using volatile liquid?

c. What do you mean by immunological products? Explain general method of preparation of toxoid.

d. Define and classify dosage form in detail.

e. Explain construction and working of silverson mixer homogeniser.

f. Give two examples of each:

    i. Disintegrating agent   iii. Plasticizer

    ii. Lubricant

Q 4. Solve any _four_ of the following:

a. Explain construction and working of fluidized bed dryer.

b. Define aerosol. Explain two-phase and three-phase system.

c. Give principle of filtration processes. Explain working of sintered glass filter.

d. What is aseptic technique? Give various sources of contamination? How are aseptic conditions maintained?

e. In what proportion 35%, 25% and 10% ointment are mixed to get 20% ointment?

f. Explain elutriation method of size separation.

Q 5. Solve any _four_ of the following:

a. Explain the factors affecting the rate of filtration according to "Darcy's law".

b. Describe in brief (any *three*):
   i. Asavas
   ii. Bhasmas
   iii. Rasas
   iv. Ksharas
   v. Ghritas

c. Give composition of any three types of glasss used as material for making a container.

d. Calculate the quantity of sodium chloride required to prepare 8 floz of 10% solution.

e. Explain the process of vacuum distillation.

f. Write a short note on continuous hot extraction.

Q 6. Solve any *four* of the following:

a. What are effervescent granules? How are they prepared?

b. Explain construction and working of ball mill.

c. What do you mean by angle of repose? How is it measured? State its importance.

d. Define and classify immunity.

e. Explain the working of single punch tablet machine.

f. Explain various steps involved in sugar coating of tablet.

Summer Examination 2004
D Pharm First Year
Pharmaceutics I

Q 1. Solve any *five* of the following:

a. Give the ideal characteristics of tablets (any *four*).

b. Define the following terms:
   i. Size separation
   ii. Sieve number

c. How will you prepare 400 ml of 45 percent alcohol from 95 percent alcohol?

d. Give the objectives of 'mixing'.

e. Define the following terms:
   i. Slurry
   ii. Filter media
   iii. Filter cake
   iv. Filtrate

f. Give the advantages and disadvantages of alcohol as a solvent.

g. Give a brief account of thermal resistance of microorganisms.

Q 2. Answer any *four* of the following:

a. Describe the construction and working of the 'disintegrator'.

b. What are the factors which affect the size reduction of drugs?

c. Define the term "clarification". Give the factors affecting rate of filtration.

d. Draw a well labelled diagram of "metafilter".

e. Define the term "capsule". Give at least three merits and demerits of capsule.

f. Describe in brief processing of "soft gelatin capsule".

Q 3. Answer any *four* of the following:

a. Describe in brief wet granulation method.

b. Give the merits and demerits of "liquid dosage forms".

c. Classify the different method of sterilisation.

d. Define the term "pharmacopoeia". Give the salient features of the latest edition of Pharmacopoeia of India.

e. What are the requirements of rubber used as packaging material?

f. What are isotonic solutions? Define hypertonic, hypotonic and paratonic solutions.

Q 4. Answer any *four* of the following:

a. Describe in brief "disintegration test" used for enteric coated tablets.

b. Give the gradation of powders as per the latest edition of Indian pharmacopoeia.

c. Give the merits and demerits of plastic containers.

d. Define "maceration". Name the various types of maceration processes.

e. Describe in brief the construction and working of a fluidised bed dryer.

f.   i. Why are horses selected for preparation of diphtheria antitoxin?

    ii. Explain in brief one method used for concentration and refinement of diphtheria antitoxin.

    iii. Give the therapeutic dose of diphtheria antitoxin.

Q 5. Answer any *four* of the following:

a. What is 'sterilisation'? How does sterilisation differ from disinfection?

b. How will you separate two immiscible liquids in laboratory?

c. Define the term 'immunity'. Classify the official vaccines.

d. Describe in brief with suitable examples:

i. Bhasmas	iii. Asavas
ii. Anjana	iv. Churnas

e. Define the term 'tablet'. What percentage deviation in weight allowed in IP for tablets weighing.

500 mg, 300 mg, 200 mg, 100 mg and 250 mg

f. Suggest one instrument/equipment for the following operations:
    i. For mixing of an ointment ingredients
    ii. For drying of a thermolabile material
    iii. For making sterile eyedrops
    iv. For distillation of two miscible liquids
    v. For sterilisation of oily injections
    vi. For sterilisation of surgical dressings
    vii. For preparation of purified water.

Q 6. Answer any *four* of the following:

a. Define the term "evaporation". Describe at least five factors which affect evaporation of a liquid.
b. Draw a well-labelled diagram of "evaporating still".
c. Define the following terms:
    i. Distillation   iii. Condenser
    ii. Still   iv. Receiver
d. Define the term "drying". Give the applications of drying.
e. Give in brief the construction and working of moist heat sterilizer.
f. Explain the principle of working of ball mill.

Winter Examination 2004
D Pharm First Year
Pharmaceutics I

Q 1. Attempt any *five* of the following:

a. Define 'drug' and 'dosage forms' with two examples for each.
b. Give 'classification of dosage forms'.
c. Name 'a special feature' of at least four 'Novel Drug Delivery Systems' with an application of each.
d. Define the term 'metrology'. How many parts of 85%, 65%, 45% and 25% alcohol should be mixed, to get 55% alcohol?
e. What are 'paratonic solutions'? What will be the effect of 'hypotonic solution in large volume' on blood cells, if injected? Why?
f. Define and differentiate between 'antitoxins' and 'toxoids'.
g. Define and differentiate between 'active immunity' and 'passive immunity'.

Q 2. Answer any *four* of the following:

a. Draw a well labelled diagram for 'aerosol packaging'.
b. Name the four mechanisms of 'size reduction'. Give and explain an example of mill based on 'impact and attrition'.

c. What are 'official standards for powders'? Give the 'principle of sedimentation method' for size separation.

d. Draw a well labelled diagram and describe the working and advantages of 'fluid energy mill'.

e. Draw a well labelled diagram of 'cyclone separator' and describe its working and applications.

f. Give a brief account of 'thermal resistance of microorganisms'.

Q 3. Answer any *four* of the following:

a. Give the account of the 'Indian pharmacopoeia' publications in chronological sequence with 'a special feature' for each one.

b. Explain the 'theory of filtration'. What are 'sintered glass filters'? Differentiate the terms 'filtration' and 'clarification'.

c. Draw a well labelled diagram to describe working and disadvantages of 'filter candle'.

d. Draw a well labelled diagram of 'metafilter'. Give its advantages.

e. Draw a well labelled diagram of a 'Soxhlet's extractor'. How it works for 'continuous hot extraction' in preparation of 'tinctures' and 'extracts'?

f. Define and explain the processes 'maceration' and 'percolation'. How are these processes 'modified' to get maximum results?

Q 4. Answer any *four* of the following:

a. Explain the mechanism of 'mixing' of 'solid powders'. What is 'demixing'?

b. Draw a well labelled diagram of 'silverson mixer homogeniser'. Describe its working and advantage.

c. Draw a well labelled diagram of 'triple roller mill'. Describe its working and applications.

d. What is 'aseptic technique'? Why is it most important in manufacture of 'immunological products'?

e. Give in brief the construction and working of moist heat sterilization.

f. What is 'sterilization by radiation'? Give its applications.

Q 5. Answer any *four* of the following:

a. When does 'distillation under reduced pressure" become essential? Draw a well labelled diagram of 'vacuum steel' to explain its working.

b. Describe with diagram, the construction and working of 'fluidised-bed dryer'.

c. What is 'lyophilization'? Describe the principle of 'freeze dryer' and give its application.

  d. Define 'sterilization'. Classify the methods of sterilization. What are applications of 'gaseous sterilization'? Give any two.

  e. What are desirable characteristics of 'containers and closures' in 'packaging of pharmaceuticals'? Give any seven characteristics.

  f. How will you prepare 'one ounce of strong potassium permanganate solution', out of which, when 5 ml diluted to 300 ml will produce 1 in 500 solution (w/v) for washing gums and teeth?

Q 6. Answer any *four* of the following:

  a. What is 'sieving'? How does IP define No. 10 sieve? What are ideal characteristics of sieve according to IP?

  b. What are the requirements for 'satisfactory compressed tablets'? Name and explain meaning of 'various defects' found in tablets.

  c. Name various types of 'tablet excipients' with their functions in 'tableting'.

  d. Explain the terms 'film coating', 'enteric coating' and 'micro-encapsulation', with their significance in pharmacy with one material for each.

  e. Define and differentiate 'hard gelatin' and 'soft gelatin' capsules.

  f. What is difference between 'purified water', 'water for injection' and 'sterile water for injection'. How is 'distilled water, prepared continuously'?

Summer Examination 2005
D Pharm First Year
Pharmaceutics I

Q 1. Solve any *ten* of the following:

  a. Enlist four methods of size separation of powder.

  b. Differentiate between maceration of organised and unorganised drug.

  c. Enlist different mechanisms of size reduction.

  d. Define pasteurization. Enlist methods for pasteurization.

  e. Give various steps involved in wet granulation of material.

  f. Differentiate between sterilisation and disinfection.

  g. What do you mean by hermetically sealed container?

  h. Give classification of immunological preparations.

  i. Define isotonic solutions. What will be the effect if hypotonic solution is injected?

  j. Define antiadherents and glidants giving one example of each.

  k. Draw diagrams of two types of condenser.

l. Differentiate between arista and asava.

m. Enlist four methods for prefiltration treatment of slurry.

n. Define conduction and convection heat processes.

Q 2. Solve any *four* of the following:

a. Explain with diagram, filtration under reduced pressure.

b. Describe in detail the test of sterility.

c. Explain sedimentation method of size separation.

d. Explain construction and working of freeze dryer. Give its applications.

e. Explain the factors affecting selection of extraction process.

f. Describe with suitable diagram, apparatus for dissolution test of tablet.

Q 3. Solve any *four* of the following:

a. Enlist various types of plastic materials used for packaging the product.

b. Explain construction and working of fluid energy mill.

c. Describe with neat labelled diagram working of filter press.

d. Explain various difficulties in filling the capsule.

e. Write history of Indian pharmacopoeia.

f. Draw diagrams of three types of mixing equipment.

Q 4. Solve any *four* of the following:

a. Explain:
   i. Haemolysis   ii. Paratonic solution

b. Draw a well-labelled diagram of "evaporating still".

c. Give various sizes and shapes of hard and soft gelatin capsules.

d. Define lamination, chipping and mottling of tablet. Explain remedial measures to overcome these difficulties.

e. Draw flow chart for dry-granulation process used for compression.

f. Define the term drying. Give applications of drying.

Q 5. Solve any *four* of the following:

a. Explain with neat labelled diagram preparation of sterile water for injection using water still.

b. Describe various factors affecting evaporation.

c. Define:
   i. Coarse powder   iii. Very fine powder
   ii. Moderately fine powder

d. From 1 in 400 solution of potassium permanganate, prepare 100 ml of 1 in 5000 solution.

e. Explain construction and working of cyclone separator.

f. Give merits and demerits of rubber as a material for closure.

Q 6. Solve any *four* of the following:

a. Find the proportion of boric acid required to make a solution isotonic with tear.

b. Differentiate between single punch and rotary tablet machine.

c. Explain with the help of neat labelled diagram working of hot air oven.

d. Describe in detail various types of "tablets for solution".

e. Define the following with one example (any *three*):

    i. Anjana   iv. Churna

    ii. Gutika   v. Arka

    iii. Sattva

f. In what proportion 30%, 20% and 10% hydrochloric acid solutions are mixed to get 15% hydrochloric solution?

Winter Examination 2005
D Pharm First Year
Pharmaceutics I

Q 1. Attempt any *ten* of the following:

a. What are pharmacopoeia? Why are they revised regularly?

b. State the importance of size reduction in pharmacy (any *four*).

c. State how liniments differ from lotions.

d. Define "evaporation", discuss three factors affecting rate of evaporation.

e. What are "galenicals"? State the different methods for preparing galanicals.

f. Define homogenisation and state its importance in pharmacy.

g. What are the requirements of "eyedrops" (standards)? (Any *four*).

h. State four differences between hard and soft gelatin capsules.

i. State the ideal qualities of granules for manufacturing tablets.

j. Which factors are taken into account while selecting a filter medium?

k. State the difference between vaccines and sera.

l. Define sterilization and give the methods of sterilization.

m. Define isotonic and paratonic solutions.

n. Why is glycerin used as a base in the preparation of throat paints?

o. Give the principle of lyophilisation.

Q 2. Answer any *four* of the following:

a. Give the construction and working of a hammer mill.

b. Give the important features of IP 1985.

  c. Discuss the process of reserved percolation process stating its advantages.

  d. State the difference between maceration and maceration with adjustment of volume.

  e. Give the construction and working of a blender used for mixing of dry powders in capsule manufacturing.

  f. Give the gradation of powder according to IP.

Q 3. Answer any *four* of the following:

  a. Give the construction and working of evaporating still.

  b. Explain the principle of steam distillation and give its application in pharmacy.

  c. Discuss sustained release dosage forms, with their advantages over traditional dosage forms.

  d. Give the construction and working of a still used for preparation of distilled water.

  e. What qualities the powder to be filled in hard gelatin capsules should possess?

  f. How do you evaluate tablets as per IP 1996? Mention disintegration time for uncoated tablets.

Q 4. Answer any *four* of the following:

  a. Give the processing stages involved in the manufacturing of tablets.

  b. What is microencapsulation? State the methods of microencapsulation.

  c. Give the construction and working of filter press.

  d. Which precautions are required to be taken for safe and effective handling of:
     i. Autoclave
     ii. Hot air oven

  e. Discuss in brief the gaseous sterilization using ethylene oxide.

  f. What are immunological products? Give their classification with one example for each class.

Q 5. Answer any *four* of the following:

  a. Give the general method of preparation for a killed bacterial vaccines. Give two examples.

  b. Calculate the quantity of sodium chloride required to prepare 500 ml of solution isotonic with blood.

  c. Give the construction and working of a cyclone separator.

  d. What are aseptic techniques? What precautions are taken for aseptic work?

e. Discuss glass as a material for making containers with advantages and disadvantages.

f. What qualities the solvent should possess to be used in extraction?

Q 6. Answer any *four* of the following:

a. Give the theory of liquid mixing.

b. What advantages the solid dosage forms have over the liquid dosage forms?

c. Give special applications of capsules.

d. Discuss tablet defects and suggest remedies to overcome the defects.

e. State the:
   i. Importance of size reduction in solid mixing.
   ii. Importance of imbibition in percolation.

f. What quantities of solute are required to be dissolved to obtain 1% solutions measuring:
   i. 110 minims   iii. 1 pint
   ii. 1 fluid ounce

Summer Examination 2006
D Pharm First Year
Pharmaceutics I

Q 1. Attempt any *five* of the following:

a. What is the principle behind distillation under reduced pressure?

b. What do you mean by immunisation?

c. Give the metric equivalents of the following:
   i. One pint   iii. One teaspoonfull
   ii. One fluid drachm   iv. 15 Grains

d. What is elutrition process?

e. Name various types of closures used.

f. Explain the function and properties of "filter aids" with suitable example.

g. Draw a labelled diagram of Soxhlet's extractor.

Q 2. Answer any *four* of the following:

a. What is the characteristic feature of third edition of IP? When it was published?

b. Draw a well-labelled diagram of silversons mixer homogeniser. Give its advantages and disadvantages.

c. What is the requirements of rubber used as packaging material.

d. Define and classify tablets. Mention official and nonofficial standards for tablets.

e. Explain construction and working of triple roller mill.
f. Write short notes on any two:
   i. Enteric coating   iii. Hard gelatin capsule
   ii. National formulary

Q 3. Answer any *four* of the following:

a. Explain principle of freez drying. Describe the process in brief.
b. What are vaccines? How is BCG vaccine prepared?
c. Differentiate between any two:
   i. Exotoxins and endotoxins
   ii. Filtration and classification
   iii. Natural and naturally accquired immunity.
d. Why is it necessary to coat the tablets? Name different methods used for it? Explain film coating.
e. How are hard gelatin capsules filled and sealed using capsule filling machine?
f. What is aseptic technique? State its importance.
   Give the precautions for safe and effective handling of sterilisation equipments.

Q 4. Answer any *four* of the following:

a. Define the term "dosage form". Classify liquid dosage forms.
b. What is reserved percolation process? How is it carried out?
c. Calculate the percentage of sodium chloride necessary to make an injection containing 2% procaine hydrochloride ISO-osmotic with blood plasma.
d. Define:
   i. Size reduction   iii. Immunity
   ii. Size separation   iv. Containers
e. What is the difference between 'purified water' and water for injection? How will you prepare water for injection in the laboratory?
f. What are different types of vaccines? Describe briefly the method of preparation of 'diphtheria antitoxin".

Q 5. Answer any *four* of the following:

a. What do you mean by term microencapsulation?
   Describe the various techniques used for the same.
b. Describe the various stages in sugar coating of tablets.
c. Give the construction, working and application of filter candle.
d. Write advantages and disadvantages of tray dryer processes.
e. Explain the theory of fractional distillation.
f. Write a note on "digestion processes" of extraction.

Q 6. Answer any *four* of the following:

a. Describe in brief:
   i. Aristas   ii. Asavas
b. Give in brief the various steps involved in the manufacturing of compressed tablets.
c. Give the construction and working of cyclone separator.
d. Describe the various equipments used for semi-solid mixing.
e. Explain the various factors which affect the size reduction of drugs.
f. Calculate the number of grains required to make 8 or a 4 percent solution and label with direction for preparing a quart of a 1 in 2000 solution.

Winter Examination 2006
D Pharm First Year
Pharmaceutics I

Q 1. Answer any *five* of the following:

a. Enlist any four methods of size separation of powder.
b. Why is it necessary to maintain the isotonicity of parenterals?
c. Name various types of closures used.
d. Write in brief note on water for injection.
e. Differentiate between maceration and infusion.
f. Define dosage forms and classify them.
g. How many parts of 60% and 40% alcohol required to prepare 50% of alcohol?

Q 2. Answer any *four* of the following:

a. Discuss the composition of glass.
b. Discuss the mechanism of mixing.
c. Discuss the working of closed circuit mill.
d. Define capsule and discuss the excipients used in manufacturing of capsules.
e. Discuss the construction and working of fluid energy mill.
f. Discuss the processing problems of tablets.

Q 3. Answer any *four* of the following:

a. Discuss the principle, construction and working of autoclave.
b. Explain soxhelation.
c. Classify and explain oral cavity tablet.
d. Discuss the theory of filtration. What are sintered glass filters and differentiate the terms filtration and clarification.

e. What are vaccines? Write the preparation of BCG vaccine.

f. Discuss the theory, apparatus and application of fractional distillation.

Q 4. Solve any *four* of the following:

a. Discuss the process involved in dry granulation method.

b. Discuss the steps involved in sugar coating tablets.

c. Discuss the factors affecting rate of evaporation.

d. How many parts of 90%, 80%, 60% and 50% alcohol be mixed to obtain 70% alcohol, 500 ml.

e. Define size reduction.

f. Discuss double maceration process.

Q 5. Solve any *four* of the following:

a. Define filtration and clarification. Discuss factors affecting rate of filtration.

b. Explain the official grades of powders.

c. Discuss the evaluation tests for tablets.

d. Discuss the various types of containers used in packaging of pharmaceuticals.

e. Explain briefly tray dryer.

f. Define sterilization and classify it and discuss dry heat sterilization.

Q 6. Solve any *four* of the following:

a. Explain the construction and working of silverson mixer homogenizer.

b. Define immunity. Discuss active and passive immunity.

c. Discuss the salient features of third and fourth edition of Indian pharmacopoeia.

d. Find the proportion of procaine hydrochloride which will yield a solution iso-osmotic with blood plasma. (Given: FP of a 1% w/v solution of procaine hydrochloride is $-0.122°C$.

e. Explain various types of containers used in pharmaceuticals.

f. Explain briefly lyophilisation.

Summer Examination 2007
D Pharm First Year
Pharmaceutics I

Q 1. Solve any *ten* of the following:

a. Differentiate between syrup and elixirs.

b. Why should powders be converted to granules before compression into tablet.

    c. Why is glycerin added to throat paints?

    d. What will happen if eyedrops are not isotonic?

    e. What should be the qualities of ideal rubber closures used for closing vials?

    f. Name the parts of an aerosol container. Give two examples of propellants used in aerosol formulation.

    g. Name the different mechanisms of size reduction with an example of mill of each type.

    h. What is levigation?

    i. What are the main objectives of mixing process?

    j. What are the applications of viscosity in pharmacy?

    k. Name the factors affecting rate of filtration.

    l. What are filter aids? What should be the qualities of ideal filter aid?

    m. Differentiate between maceration and infusion.

    n. What are asavas? How are they prepared?

Q 2. Solve any *four* of the following:

    a. What is immunity? What are the factors responsible for producing immunity in human beings.

    b. Explain the preparation of soft gelatin capsules.

    c. What are the advantages of tablet as a dosage form?

    d. What are enteric coated tablets? How are they prepared?

    e. Which are the different machines used for compression of tablets. Name the major parts of single punch tablet machine.

    f. What are granulating agents used in tablet making?

Q 3. Solve any *four* of the following:

    a. Explain with a neat labelled diagram the working of autoclave.

    b. Define coarse powder and fine powder.

    c. Explain the various factors affecting rate of evaporation.

    d. What are implants? Describe them.

    e. Calculate the quantity of dextrose, required to prepare 500 ml of 0.6% w/v solution.

    f. Differentiate between active and passive immunity.

Q 4. Solve any *four* of the following:

    a. Write qualities of an ideal container of packing pharmaceutical products? Name the materials used for making them.

    b. What is the composition of the shell of hard gelatin capsules? How should capsules be stored?

    c. Enlist the standards for pharmacopoeial sieves. Explain the sieving method of size separation.

d. Name the types of mixtures formed in mixing process. Write working of triple roller mill and its applications.

e. Define filter media. What should be its characteristics. What are the criteria for selection of filter media.

f. Write a note on membrane filters used in filtration.

Q 5. Solve any *four* of the following:

a. Name any two solvents used for extraction process. Give their advantages and disadvantages.

b. Explain double maceration process for extraction of drugs.

c. What is the importance of imbibition process in percolation? What care has to be taken while packing a percolator?

d. Name four ayurvedic dosage forms. Write a note on bhasmas.

e. Explain the working of evaporating still with a neat labelled diagram. Give its advantages and disadvantages.

f. Explain the moist granulation process of making granules.

Q 6. Solve any *four* of the following:

a. Name the term and explain it, mentioning the Indian pharmacopoeia for storage of pharmaceuticals.

b. Write a note on water for injection IP.

c. In what proportion should 50%, 20%, 10% alcohols be mixed to get 25% alcohol.

d. Define drying process. Explain the drying of materials in a rotatory dryer.

e. Draw a labelled diagram of vertical fluidised bed dryer. Give its advantages.

f. Name the gases used for sterilization. Explain the sterilization by using ethylene oxide gas.

Winter Examination 2007
D Pharm First Year
Pharmaceutics I

Q 1. Answer any *five* of the following:

a. Define drug and dosage forms.

b. Write approx. equivalents of 1 fluid ounce, 1 teaspoonful, 1 dessertspoonful, 1 tablespoonful.

c. Write any four properties of material selected for the packaging.

d. Define filtration and clarification.

e. Define extraction and menstrum.

f. Differentiate between active and passive immunity.

g. Differentiate between sustained release and controlled release with plasma concentration vs time profile.

Q 2. Answer any *four* of the following:

a. Discuss the salient features of third and fourth edition of Indian pharmacopoeias.

b. Draw a well labelled diagram of aerosol container.

c. Write principle, merits, demerits of ball mill.

d. Define tablets and discuss the method of preparation of tablet.

e. What is autoclaving? Write principle, applications and advantages.

f. Find the concentration of sodium chloride required to make a 1.5% solution of cocaine hydrochloride iso-osmotic with blood plasma. (Given: The FP of 1% w/v of cocaine hydrochloride = − 0.09°C and FP of 1% w/v solution of sodium chloride = − 0.576°C)

Q 3. Answer any *four* of the following:

a. Draw a neat diagram of Soxhlet's apparatus and discuss its principle.

b. Discuss the excipients used in mfg of tablets with suitable examples.

c. Write the special applications of capsules.

d. Write the various sources of contamination.

e. List the equipments used in drying process. Write advantages and disadvantages of tray dryer.

f. Define distillation. Draw a well labelled diagram of simple distillation process and write the applications of simple distillation in pharmacy.

Q 4. Answer any *four* of the following:

a. Define emulsions. What are its types? And enlist the various emulsifying agents used in emulsion.

b. Explain factors affecting size reduction.

c. Write the official standards for powders.

d. Write the properties of good filter media.

e. Write the advantages, disadvantages of water and alcohol as a solvent for extraction.

f. Prepare 600 ml of 60% alcohol from 95% alcohol.

Q 5. Answer any *four* of the following:

a. Write the stages involved in sterilisation of surgical dressings.

b. Describe the manufacturing defects of tablets.

c. Discuss the maceration process for organised and unorganised drugs.

d. Describe various stages involved in sugar coating.

e. Write the BCG vaccine (freeze dried) preparation method.

f. Write the applications of viscosity in pharmacy.

Q 6. Answer any *four* of the following:

a. Write construction working of cyclone separator.

b. Write the factors which affect size reduction.

c. Write cons, working, principle of fluid energy mill.

d. Write the physical properties of particles which affect perfect mixing.

e. Why are plastic containers commonly used?

f. Draw a neat diagram of filter leaf and explain construction and working of it.

Summer Examination 2008
D Pharm First Year
Pharmaceutics I

Q 1. Answer any *ten* of the following:

a. Explain the meaning of pharmacopoeia and state its importance.

b. Define "emulsions" and state two reasons for cracking of emulsions.

c. What are isotonic solutions? State their importance in 'eye lotions'.

d. Discuss four features of an ideal pharmaceutical container.

e. State four factors affecting "size reduction".

f. State importance of "size separation" in pharmacy.

g. Explain the terms "impellers, propellers, paddles and turbines" with reference to liquid mixing.

h. State any four ideal qualities of a filter medium.

i. Define "menstrum" and state three qualities of a menstrum.

j. Define distillation and suggest a method for separation of:
   i. Volatile oils from crude drugs
   ii. Miscible liquids from their mixture

k. Explain tyndallization.

l. Why are disintegrants not added to lozenges?

m. Define capsules and classify them on the basis of their composition.

n. State the difference between vaccines and sera.

Q 2. Answer any *four* of the following:

a. Name the pharmacopoeia published by WHO and give reasons for publishing European pharmacopoeia.

b. Give the construction and working of "fluid energy mill".

    c. State seven grades of powders as defined in IP 1996 stating their size ranges.

    d. Give construction and working of "cyclone separator".

    e. Explain the mechanism of solid mixing.

    f. Define creams and ointments. State their types and explain how they differ from each other.

Q 3. Answer any *four* of the following:

    a. Give the construction and working of a "planatory mixer".

    b. Explain the percolation process with the help of processing stages.

    c. What are the advantages of multiple maceration? Give the formula for calculating volume required for first maceration in multiple maceration.

    d. Give the principle of vacuum distillation. Sketch a neat labelled diagram of a "vacuum still".

    e. Explain pills giving methods of preparation, advantages and disadvantages.

    f. What proportion of alcohol 30%, 12% and 15% be mixed to obtain 18% alcohol.

Q 4. Answer any *four* of the following:

    a. Enlist the tablet excipients and discuss diluents with examples.

    b. What advantages the compression coating has over the pan coating.

    c. Give the construction and working of the meta filter.

    d. Which official and nonofficial tests are performed to evaluate tablets?

    e. Give the construction and working of evaporating still and state the advantages.

    f. Discuss the processing of hard gelatin capsules.

Q 5. Answer any *four* of the following:

    a. Define filtration and state five factors affecting rate of filtration.

    b. Define sterilization and state the methods.

    c. Discuss UV sterilization with its applications.

    d. Explain sterilization by filtration and name two medias used.

    e. What are Novel Drug Delivery Systems? How do they differ from traditional dosage forms?

    f. Give the construction and working of FBD.

Q 6. Answer any *four* of the following:

    a. Discuss "enemas" as dosage forms.

    b. Explain continuous hot percolation with the help of apparatus used.

c. Define the terms, disinfectants, immunity, vaccines, sera, antigens and toxoids.

d. How do you prepare and store diphtheria antitoxin.

e. Give the construction and working of Stoke's still.

f. Discuss rubber as a material for making closures.

Winter Examination 2008
D Pharm First Year
Pharmaceutics I

Q 1. Answer any *five* of the following:

a. Define "drug" and "dosage form".

b. What is sieve number? Give official grades of powders.

c. Why are tablets coated?

d. Define "metrology". Name the various systems of weights and measures followed in pharmacy.

e. Define isotonic solution. What will be the effect if hypertonic solution is injected?

f. How are ayurvedic dosage forms are classified? Give their examples.

g. What are the various precautions necessary to be taken while placing the material in a hot air oven?

Q 2. Answer any *four* of the following:

a. Write merits and demerits of solid dosage forms and discuss the method of preparation of soft gelatin capsule by rotary machine.

b. How many parts of 90%, 80%, 60% and 40% alcohol should be mixed so as to obtain alcohol of 70% strength, 500 ml?

c. Describe sedimentation method of size separation.

d. Discuss the working of filter press with a neat diagram.

e. Discuss the various types of tablet excipients with their functions in tableting.

f. Describe "disintegration test" for tablets.

Q 3. Answer any *four* of the following:

a. Describe salient feature of third and fourth edition of Indian pharmacopoeia.

b. Explain with the help of a diagram the various parts of aerosol packaging.

c. Discuss the various factors which affect the size reduction of drugs.

    d. Describe the planetary mixer.

    e. Define:

       i. Asava

      ii. Arista

     iii. Bhasma

     iv. Anjana

    f. Define sterilisation and classify methods of sterilisation, and discuss the principle and working of hot air oven.

Q 4. Answer any *four* of the following:

    a. Describe the various factors which affect evaporation of a liquid.

    b. Describe fractional distillation process.

    c. Name the various equipments used in drying. Explain working of fluidized bed dryer.

    d. Describe working of autoclave with a diagram.

    e. Define suspension and discuss the suspending agent used in preparation of suspension.

    f. What is multiple maceration? Discuss double maceration process.

Q 5. Answer any *four* of the following:

    a. Define vaccines. Explain the process of preparation of BCG vaccine.

    b. From 1 in 400 solution of potassium permanganate, prepare 100 ml of 1 in 5000 solution.

    c. Define tablets. Name different types of tablets and discuss the principle of sustained and controlled release tablets.

    d. Explain sterilisation by filtration.

    e. Give a brief account of filter media used for filtration.

    f. How will you separate two immiscible liquids in the laboratory? Make a labelled sketch of the apparatus used in the laboratory.

Q 6. Answer any *four* of the following:

    a. Discuss sugar coating of tablets.

    b. Define immunity and discuss the active and passive immunity.

    c. Describe the working of fluid energy mill with the help of a neat diagram.

    d. What are the different types of containers used in pharmaceutical packaging?

    e. Describe the process of simple percolation used in the preparation of tinctures.

    f. Describe with diagram, the construction and working of triple roller mill.

Summer Examination 2009
D Pharm First Year
Pharmaceutics I

Q 1. Answer any *five* of the following:

a. Why tablet dosage forms are most popular?

b. Define 'immunity' and 'immunisation'.

c. Differentiate between 'sterilisation' and 'disinfection'.

d. Define 'size separation' and 'sieve number'.

e. Define 'pharmacopoeia'. Why 'International pharmacopoeia' is published by WHO?

f. Give the importance of dosage forms.

g. Suggest an instrument for the following operations:

   i. For drying of a thermolabile material

   ii. For making sterile eyedrops

   iii. For sterilisation of surgical dressings

   iv. For preparing pharmaceutical suspensions of particle size less than one micron.

Q 2. Answer any *four* of the following:

a. Define 'aerosols'. Classify aerosols. Give advantages of aerosols.

b. Describe the different types of glass used for the making of containers.

c. Give the principle, construction and working of 'hammer mill'.

d. Give the factors which affect the size reduction of drugs.

e. Draw a well labelled diagram of 'cyclone separator'. Give its merits.

f. Find the concentration of sodium chloride required to make 1% solution of cocaine hydrochloride isotonic with blood plasma. (Freezing point of 1% w/v solution of sodium chloride is $-0.576°C$ and that of cocaine HCl is $-0.09°C$.)

Q 3. Answer any *four* of the following:

a. Explain in detail the various grades of powders official in the pharmacopoeia.

b. How does the elutriation method help in the size separation of powder? Give the merits of this method.

c. Define 'mixing'. Discuss the construction and working of planetary mixer.

d. Give the applications of 'viscosity' and 'surface tension' in pharmacy.

e. What are the objectives of 'mixing'? What are the physical properties which affect the perfect mixing of powders?

f. How will you prepare 8 oz of 60% alcohol from 95% alcohol?

Q 4. Answer any *four* of the following:

a. Define:
   i. Filtration
   ii. Filtrate
   iii. Filter medium and
   iv. Filter cake

b. Explain the construction and working of a 'plate and frame filter press'.

c. Define 'evaporation'. Describe the construction and working of evaporating pan with a neat diagram.

d. What is percolation? Explain in brief the various stages involved in carrying out official percolation process.

e. Give the applications of simple distillation. What is the principle of fractional distillation?

f. How many parts of 60%, 45% and 75% alcohol be mixed to get 50% alcohol?

Q 5. Answer any *four* of the following:

a. How distillation of two immiscible liquids is carried out?

b. Draw a well-labelled diagram of 'Soxhlet's apparatus'. What are the limitations of soxhlation method?

c. Describe in brief the construction and working of a fluidized bed dryer.

d. What is chemical sterilisation? Which chemicals are used for this process?

e. Give the principle and working of the equipment used for moist heat sterilisation.

f. Define:
   i. Drying
   ii. Lyophilisation
   iii. Sterilisation
   iv. Bactericide

Q 6. Answer any *four* of the following:

a. Classify tablets.

b. Mention official and nonofficial standards for tablets. Describe in brief weight variation test for tablets.

c. Give the characteristics of an ideal tablet.

d. Describe in brief processing of 'hard gelatin capsule'.

e. Differentiate between—'active immunity' and 'passive immunity'.

f. Discuss in brief the procedure for preparation of BCG vaccine. Give its dose, storage and uses.

Summer Examination 2010
D Pharm First Year
Pharmaceutics I

Q 1. Answer any *five* of the following:

a. What do you mean by dosage from? Why different dosage forms are required?

b. What is official and non-official compendia?

c. What do you mean by tamper resistant packaging?

d. Define impact and attrition.

e. Draw a neat labelled diagram of Soxhlet extractor.

f. Give meaning of well closed container and tightly closed container as per I.P.

g. Define immunization.

Q 2. Answer any *four* of the following:

a. Define 'size reduction'. Give importance of size reduction in pharmacy.

b. Give principle, construction and working of "Ball mill".

c. Define 'sieve number'. Give official gradation of powders.

d. Define "Isotonic solutions". What will be the effects of paratonic solution if given by I/V?

e. Give construction and working of "triple roller mill".

f. Define metrology. Prepare and supply 200 ml of 60% of alcohol from 90% alcohol.

Q 3. Answer any *four* of the following:

a. Explain principle and working of "Cyclone separator".

b. Write short note on vacuum dryer with neat diagram.

c. Enlist various manufacturing defects in tablets. Describe any two defects.

d. Draw a well labelled diagram of "Fluid energy mill" and give its principle.

e. Give classification of dosage forms with suitable examples.

f. Give in brief history of "Indian pharmacopoeia"

Q 4. Answer any *four* of the following:

a. How many tablets each containing 8.75 gr of mercuric chloride will be required to make one quart of 0.05% solution?

b. What is package and packaging? Give qualities of a "Good container".

c. Write on 'Flaking' and 'Weathering' of glass.

d. Draw a well labelled diagram of laboratory scale "steam distillation apparatus".

e. Define mixing. Describe various factors affecting perfect mixing of powder.

f. Describe "Slugging method" for manufacture of tablets.

Q 5. Answer any *four* of the following:

a. Define filtration and clarification. Describe briefly the factors which affect rate of filtration by Darcy's Law.

b. Write short note on "Metafilter"

c. Write short note on "Multiple maceration".

d. Enlist Ayurvedic dosage forms. Give difference between Asava and Arista.

e. What is evaporation? Describe factors affecting rate of evaporation.

f. Define drying. Give applications of drying in pharmacy.

Q 6. Answer any *four* of the following:

a. Define:
  i. Sterilization
  ii. Disinfectants
  iii. Antiseptics

b. Define tablets. How "Uniformity of weight" test is performed on tablets?

c. Differentiate between hard gelating capsule and soft gelating capsule.

d. Write on excipients used in filling capsule.

e. Define immunity. Differentiate between active immunity and passive immunity.

f. How many parts of 90%, 80%, 60% and 40% be mixed to obtain 70% alcohol?

Winter Examination 2010
D Pharm First Year
Pharmaceutics I

Q 1. Answer any *five* of the following:

a. Give four examples of monophasic liquid dosage forms.

b. Name the different types of materials used for making of containers.

c. Name the different methods of size reduction.

d. What does the term "perfect mixing" mean?

e. Define the term "filtrate".

f. What are the various ingredients used in the preparation of soft gelatin capsules?

g. Define the term "immunity".

Q 2. Answer any *four* of the following:

a. Give in brief the method of preparation of rabies vaccine.

b. How will you differentiate between a hard gelating capsule and soft gelatin capsule?

c. Classify the different methods of sterilization.

d. Explain the theory of fractional distillation.

e. Describe the various factors which affect evaporation.

f. Explain with the help of a neat diagram of Triple roller mill.

Q 3. Answer any *four* of the following:

a. Describe the construction, working of cyclone separator along with a neat sketch.

b. Explain the various factors which affect the size reduction of drugs.

c. Draw a well labelled diagram of aerosol packaging.

d. Calculate the percentage of sodium chloride required to make a 1% solution of hyoscine hydrobromide iso-osmotic with body fluids. The sodium chloride equivalent of 1% hyoscine hydrobromide 0.12.

e. Describe novel drug delivery system.

f. Give in brief the various steps involved in the manufacturing of tablets.

Q 4. Answer any *four* of the following:

a. Discuss the various factors responsible for producing the immunity in human beings.

b. Draw a well labelled diagram of hand operated capsule filling machine.

c. Explain the construction and working of a autoclave.

d. Differentiate between 'purified water' and water for injection'. What are applications of distillation in pharmacy?

e. Write a short note on evaporating pan.

f. Find the concentration of sodium chloride required to make a 1% solution of cocaine hydrochloride iso-osmotic with blood plasma. The freezing-point of a 1% w/v solution of cocaine hydrochloride is $-0.090°C$.

Q 5. Answer any *four* of the following:

a. Write the merits and demerits of plastic containers.

b. Draw a well labelled diagram of ball mill.

c. What are the qualities of an ideal filter aid? Describe the filter candle.

d. Write a short note on soxhelation.

e. What do you mean by distillation under reduced pressure? Explain with a neat sketch the working of the apparatus employed for the purpose of distillation under reduced pressure for laboratory scale.

f. Describe tray dryer.

Q 6. Answer any *four* of the following:

a. Mention the common defects which can occur in compressed tablets. How can such defects removed?

b. What are the various test recommended by the I.P. for evaluation of capsules?

c. Differentiate between active immunity and passive immunity.

d. Write briefly what you know about "Tyndallisation".

e. Draw a well labelled diagram of fluidized bed dryer.

f. Name any *one* marketed preparation of following:

i. Anjan	ii. Arkas
iii. Aristas	iv. Bhasmas
v. Churnas	vi. Gutikas
vii. Rasas	

Summary Examination 2011
D Pharm First Year
Pharmaceutics I

Q 1. Answer any *ten* of the following:

a. Define drug and dosage forms.

b. Name various types of closures used.

c. List any four important advantages of tablets.

d. List any four qualities of good container.

e. Define pharmacopoeia. List official books used in India.

f. List any for methods used for size reduction.

g. Write the advantages of elutrition method.

h. Write the main objectives of mixing.

i. Write any four properties of good filter media.

j. Write the advantages of alcohol as solvent for extraction.

k. Write the disadvantages of evaporating pan.

l. Write any four applications of simple distillation.

m. List any four equipment used in drying process.

n. Why formaldehyde is not used as sterilisation purposes in gaseous sterilisation method.

Q 2. Answer any *four* of the following:

a. Draw a well labelled diagram of aerosol container.

b. Write the official standards for powders.

c. Describe the history of Indian pharmacopoeia.

d. Write the difference between hard gelatin and soft gelatin capsules.

e. Draw a well labelled diagram of Silversons mixter homogenizer. Give its advantages and disadvantages.

f. List advantages of plastic as packaging material.

Q 3. Answer any *four* of the following:

a. List the applications of viscosity in pharmacy.

b. Explain various factors which affects rate of filtration.

c. Explain the simple maceration process.

d. Write the applications of drying in industry.

e. Write the advantages of dry heat sterilization.

f. Why tablets are coated?

Q 4. Answer any *four* of the following:

a. List the various excipients used in Tablets with suitable example.

b. Draw a well labelled diagram of Soxhlet's Apparatus.

c. Write the advantages and disadvantages of capsule.

d. Explain the manufacturing defects in tablet manufacturing.

e. List down the evaluation test carried out on Tablets. Explain friability test.

f. Define immunity and explain types of immunity.

Q 5. Answer any *four* of the following:

a. Why soda lime glass is not used for the parenteral preparations?

b. Name the method used for sterilisation of following substances:
   i. Surgical hand gloves   ii. Injectables
   iii. Hospital wards

c. Explain construction and working of cyclone separator.

d. Give the factors which affect size reduction.

e. Define aseptic technique. What are the various sources of contamination?

f. What are the precautions to be taken while handling eye drops?

Q 6. Answer any *four* of the following:

a. Define emulsions. What are types of emulsions?

b. Why yellow soft paraffin is used in ophthalmic pren.?

c. How are hard gelating capsule filled and sealed using capsule filling machine?

d. How BCG vaccine is prepared by Freeze drying method?

e. In what proportion should 20% HCl and 10% HCl mixed to get 15% HCl?

f. Find out proportion of procaine HCl which will yield Sol^n iso-osomotic with blood plasma.

Given. F.P. of 1% P. HCl = 0.122°C.

Winter Examination 2011
D Pharm First Year
Pharmaceutics I

Q 1. Answer any *eight* of the following:

a. Enlist methods of size reduction.

b. Differentiate between organized and unorganized drug.

c. Give various steps involved in dry granulation method.

d. Enlist methods of size separation.

e. Classify immunity.

f. Define osmosis, isotonic solution.

g. Define dosage form and classify it.

h. Write various types of closures.

i. List any four equipment used in drying.

j. Write the advantages of alcohol for extraction.

k. Write any four applications of simple distillation.

l. Define pharmacopoeia. List official books used in India.

Q 2. Answer any *four* of the following:

a. Discuss the working of ball mill.

b. Discuss the composition of glass.

c. Explain the mechanisms of mixing.

d. Define capsule and explain excipients used in manufacturing capsules.

e. Explain processing problems of tablets.

f. Explain the working of fluid energy mill.

Q 3. Answer any *four* of the following:

a. Discuss the principle and working of autoclave.

b. Explain the method of soxhelation.

c. Explain the classification of oral cavity tablets.

d. Explain factors affecting rate of filtration.

e. Write the preparation and application of BCG vaccine.

f. Discuss the principle and working of fractional distillation.

Q 4. Answer any *four* of the following:

a. Explain wet granulation method.

b. Explain different types of coating of tablets.

c. Explain factors affecting rate of evaporation.

d. Discuss double maceration process.

e. How many parts of 90%, 80%, 60% and 50% alcohol be mixed to obtain 70% alcohol?

f. Explain types of heat process.

Q 5. Answer any *four* of the following:

a. Explain types of mixing.

b. Explain official grades of powder.

c. Explain evaluation test of tablets.

d. Explain briefly tray dryer.

e. Discuss various types of containers used in packaging pharmaceutical products.

f. Define sterilization and classify it.

Q 6. Answer any *four* of the following:

a. Explain the working of Silverson mixer homogenizer.

b. Explain the preparation of hard gelatin and soft gelatin capsule.

c. Draw a neat labelled diagram of aerosol and give its application.

d. Explain simple maceration process.

e. Explain various methods of coating of tablets.

f. Explain briefly lyophilisation.

Summer Examination 2012
D Pharm First Year
Pharmaceutics I

Q 1. Answer any *five* of the following:

a. Give reasons, why tablets are coated.

b. Write the precautions to be taken while placing the material in hot air oven.

c. Give the importance of dosage forms.

d. Give the pharmaceutical significance of size reduction.

e. Give the difference between hard and soft gelatin cap.

f. Give the steps involved in wet granulation method.

g. Write any four factors which affect filtration rate.

Q 2. Answer any *four* of the following:

a. What precautions are taken while using eye drops?

b. In what proportion 25%, 18%, 12% alcohol should be mixed to get 15% alcohol?

c. Write the excipients used in tablets with example.

d. Write the salient features of IIIrd edition of IP.

e. Write the advantages and disadvantages of glass as a material for packing.

f. Draw a well labelled diagram of aerosol container and give its applications.

Q 3. Answer any *four* of the following:

a. Write principle, construction, working of Hammer Mill.

b. Enlist the factors affecting size reduction.

c. Draw a labelled diagram of cyclone separator and write the advantages.

d. Explain various grades of powders.

e. Give the applications of viscosity in pharmacy.

f. Write advantages of Ball Mill.

Q 4. Answer any *four* of the following:

a. Describe the factors which affect rate of the evaporation of liquid.

b. Write the applications of simple distillation in pharmacy.

c. Describe working of autoclave with diagram.

d. Describe the simple maceration process.

e. Write advantages of fluid energy mill with figure.

f. Explain working, construction of filter leaf with neat figure.

Q 5. Answer any *four* of the following:

a. Give the principle, working of FBD (Fluidized Bed Dryer).

b. Why formaldehyde is not used as sterilizing agent?

c. Explain tray dryer with advantages, disadvantages and figure.

d. Write the manufacturing defects of tablets.

e. Write the difference between active and passive immunity.

f. Discuss the preparation method of BCG vaccine with dose, storage and uses.

Q 6. Answer any *four* of the following:

a. Write the types of tablets and give disadvantages.

b. What are enteric coated tablets? Why they are coated?

c. Write the special applications of capsules.

d. Describe the Friability test apparatus of tablets.

e. Describe the hot air oven method for sterilisation.

f. Write the stages involved in sterilisation of surgical dressings.

Winter Examination 2012
D Pharm First Year
Pharmaceutics I

Q 1. Solve any *ten* of the following:

a. Define 'Pharmaceutical aid'. Mention any two types of pharmaceutical aid with one example of each.

b. Differentiate between exotoxin and endotoxin.

c. Give 'Classification of ayurvedic dosage form' with one example.

d. Define the term 'Menstrum' and 'Marc'.

e. How many grams of potassium permanganate should be required in preparing 500 ml of 1 in 1000 solution?

f. Define 'Slurry' and Filter cake'.

g. Define 'Sustained release dosage form'. Give four advantages of it.

h. What are the limitations of 'Continuous hot percolation process'?

i. Why imbibition is necessary before packing of the drug into the percolator?

j. Define 'Galenicals'. Give two examples of galenical preparations.

k. Define 'Prodrug'. Write any two applications of it.

l. Why injectable should not be stored in soda lime glass containers?

m. What are unit dose packing? Give two examples.

Q 2. Answer any *four* of the following:

a. Give the gradation of powder according to I.P.

b. Define pharmaceutical container. Give qualities of a good container.

c. Give the principle, construction and working of colloidal mill.

d. Discuss the factors affecting the rate of filtration.

e. Give the principle, method and applications of sterilization by UV radiation method.

f. Define the term 'Tablet'. Give advantages and disadvantages of it.

Q 3. Answer any *four* of the following:

a. Give construction, working and application of 'fluidized bed dryer'.

b. Define the term 'Filter aids'. Write the four qualities of an ideal filter aids.

c. What precautions are required to be taken for safe and effective handling of following:

   i. Autoclave

   ii. Hot air oven

  d. Enlist different manufacturing defects that may appear in tablets. Explain in brief any two manufacturing defects in tablets.
  e. Define the term "Immunity". What are the factors responsible for producing immunity in human beings?
  f. Define the term "Ointments". Why the white soft paraffin is not used for the preparation of ophthalmic ointments? Give the properties of an ideal ointment base.

Q 4. Answer any *four* of the following:

  a. Draw a well labelled diagram of 'Cyclone separator' and describe its working and application.
  b. With neat labelled diagram of 'Silverson homogenizer', give principle and working of it.
  c. Define the term 'Capsule'. Give at least four merits and demerits of capsule.
  d. Give the principle and working of distillation under reduced pressure, with diagram.
  e. What is meant by levigation and Elutriation? Give the advantages of elutriation process.
  f. Draw a well labelled diagram of ball mill and give its advantages and disadvantages.

Q 5. Answer any *four* of the following:

  a. Explain the method of preparation of BCG vaccine.
  b. Explain in detail "Evaporating still" with their advantages and disadvantages.
  c. Define the term 'Suspension'. Give the properties of an ideal suspension.
  d. Draw a well labelled diagram of 'Filter candle'. Give the working and disadvantages of it.
  e. Give the importance of dosage forms.
  f. Explain the moist granulation process of making granules.

Q 6. Answer any *four* of the following:

  a. Differentiate between "active immunity" and "passive immunity".
  b. Define closures. Give their types with examples.
  c. Differentiate between hard gelatin capsule and soft gelatin capsule.
  d. Explain in brief factors affecting the process of size reduction.
  e. Define the term "Filtration". Write the working of filter press with neat labelled diagram.
  f. What is meant by evaporation? Explain the factors affecting evaporation of a liquid.

Summer Examination 2013
D Pharm First Year
Pharmaceutics I

Q 1. Answer any *five* of the following:

a. Define the term:
  i. Drug   ii. Dosage forms
b. State in chronological order different edition of Indian pharmacopoeia.
c. Draw a well labelled diagram of aerosol container.
d. State difference between hard gelatine and soft gelatine capsules.
e. State what quantities of solute are required to dissolve to obtain 1% solutions measuring:
  i. 1 fluid ounce
  ii. 1 pint
f. State application of viscosity in pharmacy.
g. Draw a well labelled diagram of Soxhlet apparatus.

Q 2. Answer any *four* of the following:

a. Give the working of Double cone blender, state its application.
b. Name and explain the mill which works on principle of combined impact and attrition.
c. State official grades of powders as per Indian pharmacopoeia.
d. Explain Darcy law with respect to rate of filtration.
e. Explain the term Galenicals. Explain process of percolation with example of any one official preparation.
f. State classification of dosage forms with suitable examples.

Q 3. Answer any *four* of the following:

a. Define tablets and classify different types of tablets.
b. Define immunity and differentiate between active and passive immunity.
c. Define capsule, state the composition of capsule shell, give merit and demerit of capsules as dosage form.
d. Explain the term sterilization, classify different methods of sterilization.   )
e. Explain in brief about 'fractional distillation'.
f. State salient features of fourth edition of Indian pharmacopoeia.

Q 4. Answer any *four* of the following:

a. How many parts of 90%, 80%, 60% and 40% alcohol should be mixed so as to obtain 70% alcohol?

b. Define:
   i. Closure
   ii. Container, state various types of closures, state various materials to be used for making closures.
c. Explain various factors affecting rate of evaporation.
d. Suggest one instrument/equipment for the following operations:
   i. For sterilization of oily injections
   ii. For sterilization of apron
   iii. For sterilization of hand gloves
   iv. For sterilization of operation theatre.
e. Explain the term Micro-encapsulation. Enlist various techniques of micro-encapsulation. State its advantages.
f. Define the following:
   i. Filtration   ii. Clarification
   iii. Filter media   iv. Filter cake
   v. Filter aid

Q 5. Answer any *four* of the following:

a. Explain the term Marc and Menstrum, state ideal properties of menstrum.
b. State construction and working of vacuum dryer.
c. State principle, construction and working of ball mill.
d. State working of cyclone separator along with its application.
e. State some special applications of capsules.
f. State and explain various mechanisms of heat transfer.

Q 6. Answer any *four* of the following:

a. Describe method of preparation of water for injection IP.
b. Describe construction, working and application of the apparatus used for moist heat sterilization.
c. State reasons for coating tablets. Explain various stages in sugar coating.
d. What are immunological products? Explain preparation method of BCG vaccine.
e. Explain construction and working of fluidized bed dryer.
f. State and explain new drug delivery system (any *three*)

Winter Examination 2013
D Pharm First Year
Pharmaceutics I

Q 1. Answer any *five* of the following:

a. Define the terms:
   i. Suspension   ii. Emulsion

b. Enlist official grades of powders. Define the term sieve no.

c. State the uses of soft-gelatin capsules.

d. Define the term:
   i. Menstruum
   ii. Marc

e. Enlist the evaluation tests for compressed tablets.

f. What are 'Aseptic techniques'

g. What are the gases used in the gaseous sterilization? What are the advantages of ethylene-oxide?

Q 2. Answer any *four* of the following:

a. Classify solid dosage forms. Write in brief about dusting powder.

b. Define the term 'Pharmacopoeia'. Write any six salient features of third edition of Indian Pharmacopoeia (1985).

c. Describe construction working of fluid energy mill.

d. State the principle, construction, working of disintegrator.

e. Enlist different methods used for size separation. Describe construction and working of 'Cyclone separator'

f. Give merits and demerits of glass as container for pharmaceutical products.

Q 3. Answer any *four* of the following:

a. How many parts of 80%, 65%, 32% and 20% alcohol to be mixed together so as to give 40% alcohol?

b. Describe various defects in tablets.

c. Define 'aerosols'. Explain with help of diagram the various parts of aerosol packaging.

d. Draw a neat labelled diagram of 'planetary mixer', state its uses.

e. Define 'Pharmaceutical containers'. What are qualities of an ideal container?

f. Draw a neat labelled diagram of 'Evaporating still'. Give its advantages and disadvantages.

Q 4. Answer any *four* of the following:

a. Draw a labelled diagram of Triple-roller mill. State its uses.

b. Define the term 'Filtration'. What are the factors which affect the rate of filtration?

c. Explain the principle, construction, working of 'Filter press'.

d. Differentiate between 'maceration of organized drugs' and 'maceration of unorganized drugs'.

e. Draw a well-labelled diagram of Soxhlet apparatus.

f. What are advantages and disadvantages of sterilization by ionizing radiation?

Q 5. Solve any *four* of the following:

a. Write in brief about common ayurvedic dosage forms.

b. What are different types of distillation? What is purified water? What is water for injection?

c. Describe construction, working of fluidised bed dryer. Write advantages and disadvantages of it.

d. What are the applications of dry heat sterilization? Describe hot air oven.

e. How are the following sterilized? Name only method:

    i. Surgical dressing   ii. Transfusion fluid

    iii. Plastic syringes   iv. Petridisthes

    v. Talc powder   vi. Insulin injection.

    vii. Aseptic area

f. Describe briefly 'Reserve percolation process'

Q 6. Answer any *four* of the following:

a. Define compressed tablet. Classify tablets.

b. Why is coating of tablets done? Enlist different methods of tablet coating. Write in brief about enteric coating.

c. Differentiate between hard Gelatin and soft Gelatin capsules.

d. Define the term immunity. Differentiate between active immunity and passive immunity.

e. Define the term vaccine. Write any one method of preparation of 'smallpox' vaccine.

f. Find the concentration of sodium chloride required to make a 1.5% solution of cocaine hydrochloride iso-osmotic with blood plasma. (Given: The freezing point of 1% w/v solution of cocaine hydrochloride is $-0.09°C$. The freezing point of 1% w/v solution of sodium chloride $-0.576°C$)

Winter Examination 2014
D Pharm First Year
Pharmaceutics I

Q 1. Answer any *ten* of the following:

a. List the different types of material used for making of the containers.

b. Enlist the methods of size reduction.

c. Define the term immunity.

d. Differentiate between organized and unorganized drugs.

e. Give the classification of dosage form.

f. In what proportion should 20% HCL be mixed with 10% HCL to obtain 15% HCL solution.

g. List the pharmacopoeias commonly used in India.

h. Write the advantages of alcohol as solvent for extraction.

i. Write the difference between hard and soft gelatin capsules.

j. Write the advantages of tablet.

k. Write the applications of simple distillation in pharmacy.

l. Write the main objectives of mixing.

Q 2. Answer any *four* of the following:

a. Explain factor affecting rate of filtration.

b. Write advantages and applications of autoclaving.

c. Write a short note on Elutriation process.

d. Explain the advantages and disadvantages of the freeze dryer.

e. Explain the limitations of soxlation with diagram.

f. Write the principle behind the distillation under reduced pressure.

Q 3. Answer any *four* of the following:

a. Write the advantages and disadvantages of plastic as a material for packaging.

b. Explain construction and working of fluid energy mill.

c. Describe the working of filter press with neat diagram.

d. Mention and explain with example the excipients used in capsules.

e. Write the history of Indian pharmacopoeia.

f. Draw a neat diagram of ball mill. Mention disadvantages of ball mill.

Q 4. Answer any *four* of the following:

a. What precautions are taken while using eye drops?

b. Define evaporation and draw a labeled diagram of evaporating still.

c. Write the special applications of capsules.

d. Enlist manufacturing defects of tablets. Explain any *two*.

e. Draw a flowchart for dry granulation process.

f. Write the applications of drying in pharmaceutical industry.

Q 5. Answer any *four* of the following:

a. What is moist heat sterilization? Write the various conditions prescribed for it.

b. Define sterilization. Why formaldehyde is not used as agent for gaseous sterilization.

c. What are aseptic techniques? Write the all possible sources for contamination.

d. Why tablets are coated? Give reasons. Mention steps involved in sugar coating.

e. Enlist the tests which are carried for evaluation of tablets.

f. How BCG vaccines (freeze dried) are prepared?

Q 6. Answer any *four* of the following:

  a. Define the followings:
    i. Anjana   ii. Churna
    iii. Arishta   iv. Ghana
  b. Explain working of hot air oven with diagram.
  c. Write the construction, working and give use of spray dryer.
  d. Write the advantages of parenteral dosage forms over solid dosage forms. What is enema?
  e. Give merits and demerits of glass as container.
  f. Draw well labelled diagram of Aerosol packaging. What do you mean by air tight container?

Summer Examination 2015
D Pharm First Year
Pharmaceutics I

Q 1. Answer any *ten* of the following:

  a. Define drugs and dosage forms with example.
  b. Name various closures used in packaging industry.
  c. Enlist four methods of size reduction.
  d. Define Aristhas and Asavas.
  e. Write any four applications of simple distillation.
  f. List any four advantages of tablets.
  g. Write the main objectives of mixing.
  h. Write any four properties of ideal container.
  i. Define pharmacopoeia. List any four books.
  j. Write the advantages of ball mill.
  k. Write the advantages of glass as a container.
  l. Formaldehyde is not used in gaseous sterilisation. Why?
  m. Write the importance of size reduction.
  n. Write the advantages of hammer mill.

Q 2. Answer any *four* of the following:

  a. Write the official standards of powders.
  b. Write the difference between hard and soft gelatin cap.
  c. List advantages of plastic as packaging material.
  d. Draw a neat diagram of silverson mixer.
  e. Write the history of Indian pharmacopoeia.
  f. Draw a well labelled diagram of aerosol container.

Q 3. Answer any *four* of the following:

  a. Give reasons. Why tablets are coated?
  b. Write the applications of drying.

c. Write the advantages of dry heat sterilisation.
d. Write the factors affecting rate of filtration.
e. Write the applications of viscosity in pharmacy.
f. What is simple maceration process?

Q 4. Answer any *four* of the following:
a. What are excipients used in tablet manufacturing?
b. Write advantages and disadvantages of capsules.
c. Give the manufacturing defects in tablet manufacturing.
d. Enlist the evaluation test for tablet. Explain any one.
e. Define immunity and explain the types of immunity.
f. Draw a neat diagram of cyclone separator.

Q 5. Answer any *four* of the following:
a. Why different dosage forms are needed?
b. Why white soft paraffin is not used in the preparation of ointments especially opthalmic ointments?
c. How BCG vaccine is prepared by freeze drying method?
d. Explain the construction and working of air separator.
e. Why soda lime glass container is not used for the parenterals?
f. In what proportion should 20% and 10% HCl is to be mixed to get 15% HCl.

Q 6. Answer any *four* of the following:
a. Name the various methods used for sterilisation: (any **two**)
   i. Hand gloves—rubber   ii. Injectables
   iii. Hospital wards.
b. Explain working and construction of ball mill.
c. What are aseptic technique? What are various sources of contamination?
d. What instructions are to be printed on opthalmic preparation?
e. Write factors affecting rate of filtration.
f. Write advantages and disadvantages of filter press.

Winter Examination 2015
D Pharm First Year
Pharmaceutics I

Q 1. Answer any *eight* of the following:
a. Enlist four methods for size reduction.
b. Define 'drug' and 'dosage form'.
c. Write the main objectives of mixing.

   d. Name any four materials used for packaging.
   e. Define 'slurry' and 'filter cake'.
   f. Why are tablets coated?
   g. Differentiate between active and passive immunity.
   h. Define 'menstruum' and state three ideal qualities of a menstrum.
   i. Why injectables should not be stored in soda lime glass containers?
   j. List any four equipments used in drying.
   k. Give steps involved in moist granulation.
   l. Define pharmacopoeia. List official books used in India.

Q 2. Answer any *four* of the following:
   a. Define sterilisation and classify methods of sterilisation.
   b. Describe construction and working of a cyclone separator with a neat diagram.
   c. How many parts of 60%, 45% and 75% alcohol should be mixed to get 50% alcohol?
   d. Explain the factors which affect size reduction of drugs.
   e. Differentiate between hard gelatin and soft gelatin capsules.
   f. Describe in brief the procedure for preparation of BCG vaccine along with its dose, storage and uses.

Q 3. Answer any *four* of the following:
   a. Draw a well-labelled diagram of soxhlet apparatus. What are the limitations of soxhletion method?
   b. Enlist different manufacturing defects that may appear in tablets. Explain in brief any two defects.
   c. Give the importance of dosage forms.
   d. Explain in detail evaporating still with its advantages and disadvantages.
   e. Differentiate between purified water and water for injection.
   f. Write the working of filter press with a neat labelled diagram.

Q 4. Answer any *four* of the following:
   a. Explain the factors affecting evaporation of a liquid.
   b. Draw a well-labelled diagram of filter candle. Give its working and disadvantages.
   c. Write advantages and disadvantages of glass as a material for packaging.
   d. Define drying. Give applications of drying in pharmacy.
   e. Describe in brief history of Indian Pharmacopoeia.
   f. Give principle and working of Silverson homogeniser with a neat labelled diagram.

Q 5. Answer any *four* of the following:

    a. Define 'aseptic technique'. What are the various sources of contamination?

    b. Give the principle and working of fluidised bed dryer.

    c. Write the special applications of capsules.

    d. State various grades of powder official in I.P.

    e. Define pharmaceutical container. Give qualities of an ideal container.

    f. Discuss working of ball mill with a neat diagram.

Q 6. Answer any *four* of the following:

    a. Draw a well-labelled diagram of aerosol container and give its advantages and disadvantages.

    b. Mention official and non-official evaluation tests for tablets. Describe weight variation test for tablets.

    c. Give applications of simple distillation. What is the principle of fractional distillation?

    d. Explain principle and working of fluid energy mill with a diagram.

    e. Describe with diagram working of autoclave.

    f. Find out the proportion of procaine HC1 which will yield solution iso-osmotic with blood plasma.

Given: F.P. of 1% procaine HC1 = –0.122°C

Summer Examination 2016
D Pharm First Year
Pharmaceutics I

Q 1. Answer any *eight* of the following:

    a. What are advantages of liquid dosage form?

    b. What are pharmacopoeias and why they are needed?

    c. Name various mechanisms of size reduction.

    d. Differentiate between hard gelatin capsule and soft gelatin capsule.

    e. Define:
        i. Capping
        ii. Lamination

    f. What are objectives of mixing?

    g. Define:
        i. Arka
        ii. Gutika

    h. Give any two applications of of fluidized bed dryer.

    i. Give any four precautions to be taken during aseptic work.

j. What are filter aids? What should be qualities of filter aids.
k. Name various types of closures.
1. Classify immunity.

Q 2. Answer any *four* of the following:

a. Give the construction and working of Silverson mixer homogeniser.
b. Discuss in brief the stepwise process of percolation used in preparation of tinctures.
c. Give the principle, construction and working of 'Ball Mill'.
d. Describe the various factors affecting size reduction.
e. Explain principle of 'Freeze drying'. Give its advantages.
f. Describe the construction and working of 'evaporating pan' with neat diagram.

Q 3. Answer any *four* of the following:

a. Describe in detail various oral cavity tablets.
b. Classify different dosage forms with examples.
c. Draw a well-labelled diagram of fluidized .bed dryer.
d. Discuss the salient features of third edition of pharmacopoeia.
e. Explain factors which affect rate of filtration by Darcy's law.
f. Define aerosols. Classify aerosols. Give formula of aerosol with example.

Q 4. Answer any *four* of the following:

a. Discuss in brief gaseous sterilization using ethylene oxide.
b. Give merits and demerits of rubber as a material for closure.
c. Explain theory of fractional distilation.
d. Discuss factors affecting evaporation.
e. Differentiate between maceration process for organised drugs and maceration for unorganised drugs.
f. Why there is need for formulation of different dosage form?

Q 5. Answer any *four* of the following:

a. What is difference between 'Purified water' and 'Water injection? How will you prepare 'Water for injection' in laboratory?
b. Describe construction and working of equipment used for moist heat sterilization.
c. In what proportion 25%, 18%, 12% alcohol should be mixed to get 15% alcohol?
d. What are various 'Novel drug delivery systems'? Explain implants.
e. Describe construction and working of double cone blender.
f. Give the method of preparation of "Smallpox vaccine" using egg.

Q 6. Answer any *four* of the following:

a. How will you prepare 4 ounces of solution so that 1 tablespoonful to 1 quart make 1 in 500 ml solution?

b. Discuss in brief disintegration test for uncoated tablet.

c. What are toxoids? Discuss general methods for preparation of toxoids.

d. Define:
   i. Sterilization
   ii. Disinfection
   Classify different methods of sterilization.

e. What are advantages of multiple maceration? Give formula for calculating volume required for double and triple maceration.

f. Explain principle, construction and working of cyclone separator.

Winter Examination 2016
D Pharm First Year
Pharmaceutics I

Q 1. Answer any *eight* of the following:

a. What is lyophilization?

b. Define the terms "phagocytosis and antibodies".

c. Enlist different filter mediums used for filtration.

d. Explain the terms :
   i. Arak
   ii. Svarasas

e. Define Emulsion.

f. Why capsules are preferred to powder?

g. Mention the application of liposomes in pharmacy.

h. Explain the importance of closures.

i. What are the different mechanism involved in the method of size reduction?

j. Draw a well-labelled diagram of "triple roller mill".

k. Give the difference between "purified water" and "water for injection".

l. Why enteric coating is given to the tablet?

Q 2. Answer any *four* of the following:

a. List the qualities of an ideal "filter aid" and state two examples of it.

b. Explain construction and working of Silverson mixer homogenizer.

c. Define "Sieve numbers" and enlist standard for sieve as per I.P.

d. Give the principle, working and application of autoclave.

e. Discuss the excipients used in filling of hard gelatin capsule with example.

f. State the salient features of the fourth edition of pharmacopoeia of India.

Q 3. Answer any *four* of the following:

a. Give the principle, working and application of "fractional distillation."

b. Define the term "clarification". Write the working of filter candle with neat diagram.

c. State and explain the stages of simple percolation.

d. Draw a well-labelled diagram of Aerosol container and state the method of Aerosol packaging.

e. List the importance of size reduction in pharmaceutical industries.

f. Explain the principle and construction of "Planetary mixer."

Q 4. Answer any *four* of the following:

a. Differentiate between maceration of "organized drug" and "unorganised drug."

b. Explain theory of Freeze drying and state its application.

c. Draw a well-labelled diagram of "Vacuum-still" and describe its theory.

d. Classify the methods of sterilisation with example.

e. State and explain the steps involved in sugar coating of tablet.

f. How many milliliters of 60% w/w syrup and 20% w/w syrup are required to prepare 300 ml of a 30% w/w syrup?

Q 5. Answer any *four* of the following:

a. Draw the well-labelled diagram of "fluidised bed dryer" (F.B.D.) and state it's disadvantage.

b. State the difference between hard gelatin and soft gelatin capsules.

c. Give the principle and working of "Fluid energy mill."

d. Explain the construction and working of cyclone sepearator.

e. Explain construction and working of "Evaporating still".

f. What do you mean by "Tyndallisation" and "Pasteurisation"? State the methods of pasteurisation.

Q 6. Answer any *four* of the following:

a. Write the reason and remedies for "Capping" of tablets.

b. Define immunity and classify it.

c. Define desiccation with two examples of dessiccant and draw a diagram of "Desiccator".

   d. State the principle, construction, working and uses of "Disintegrator".

   e. Differentiate between liniments and lotions.

   f. Give advantage and disadvantages of plastic as material for container and state its type.

Summer Examination 2017
D Pharm First Year
Pharmaceutics I

Q 1. Answer any *six* of the following:

   a. Define Pharmacopoeia. Give example.

   b. Define container and closure.

   c. What are qualities of good container?

   d. What is difference between filtration and clarification?

   e. Give application of Freeze drying.

   f. What are advantages of water as menstrum for extraction?

   g. What are advantages of evaporating still?

   h. Calculate the quality of dextrose required to prepare one quart of 5% solution.

   i. Draw a labelled diagram of double cone blender.

Q 2. Answer any *four* of the following:

   a. Define the following terms:

      i. Drug   ii. Dosage form

      iii. Excipients

   b. Define Aerosols. What are the advantages and disadvantages of Aerosols?

   c. Explain the working, advantages and disadvantages of any one mill based on the principle of combined impact and attrition.

   d. Define size reduction. What are the different factors affecting to the rate of size reduction?

   e. How many tablets, each containing 8.75 grains of mercuric chloride will be required to make one pint of 0.2% solution?

   f. Write short note on: (any **one**)

      i. Classification of liquid dosage forms

      ii. Materials used in plecutical closures

Q 3. Answer any *four* of the following:

   a. Differentiate between simple and modified maceration with example.

   b. Define capsule as a dosage form along with its advantages and disadvantages.

   c. What do you mean by enteric coated tablets? Give reasons for enteric coating.

   d. Differentiate between filtration and classification. Enlist the different factors affecting the rate of filtration.

   e. How will you prepare 330 g of dilute acetic acid from acetic acid IP.

   Given:

      i. Acetic acid IP = 33% water of acetic acid.

      ii. Dilute acetic acid = 6% water of acetic acid.

   f. Write short notes on: (any **one**)

      i. Metafilter

      ii. Additives in tablet formulation

Q 4. Answer any *four* of the following:

   a. Differentiate between hard and soft gelatin capsules with example.

   b. Define tablet as a dosage form along with advantages and disadvantages.

   c. What do you mean by reserved percolation? Enlist the different steps involved in it.

   d. Explain different steps involved in sugar coating of tablet.

   e. How will you prepare 180g of Cmehona powder containing 6% alkaloid from the three lots of powder containing 10%, 8% and 3% alkaloids.

   f. Write short note on: (any **one**)

      i. Filter aids

      ii. Ayurvedic dosage forms

Q 5. Answer any *four* of the following:

   a. Differentiate between active and passive immunity along with examples.

   b. Define microencapsulation. What are its advantages and different techniques involved in it?

   c. Define drying. What are the different factors affecting to the rate of drying?

   d. Differentiate between evaporation and distillation. Explain the working and applications of simple distillation in pharmacy.

   e. Find the cone of sodium chloride required to make 1% w/v solution of cocaine HC1 iso-osmotic with blood plasma.

   Given:

      i. F.P. of 1% w/v cocaine HC1 = $-0.09°C$

      ii. F.P. of 1% w/v sodium chloride = $-0.576°C$

   f. Write short note on: (any **one**)

      i. BCG vaccine

      ii. Silverson-mixer homogenizer

Q 6. Answer any *four* of the following:

a. Differentiate between sterilization and disinfection. Enlist the different methods of sterilization with examples.

b. Define immunity. What are the different types of immunity?

c. Define size separation. How will you grade the powders according to IP 1985?

d. Explain the objectives of mixing. Explain the different types of mixtures along with examples.

e. Find the concentration of sodium chloride required to produce a solution iso-osmotic with blood plasma.
   Given: Molecular weight of sodium chloride = 58.5 and it dissociate into 2 ions.

f. Write short note on: (any **one**)
   i. Cyclone separator
   ii. Fluidized bed dryer.